Ultrasound and the Uterus

PROGRESS IN OBSTETRIC AND GYNECOLOGICAL SONOGRAPHY SERIES

SERIES EDITOR: ASIM KURJAK

Ultrasound and the Uterus

Edited by

R. OSMERS and A. KURJAK

The Parthenon Publishing Group

International Publishers in Medicine, Science & Technology

NEW YORK LONDON

British Library Cataloguing in Publication Data
Ultrasound and the Uterus. – (Progress in Obstetric & Gynecological Sonography Series)
I. Osmers, R. II. Kurjak, Asim III. Series
618.1407543

ISBN 1-85070-613-1

Library of Congress Cataloging-in-Publication Data
Osmers, R.
Ultrasound and the uterus / R. Osmers and A. Kurjak.
p. cm. – (Progress in obstetric and gynecological sonography series : v. 2)
Includes bibliographical references and index.
ISBN 1-85070-613-1
1. Uterus–Ultrasonic imaging. I. Kurjak, Asim II. Title. III. Series. [DNLM: 1. Uterus–ultrasonography. 2. Uterine Diseases–ultrasonography. WP 141 083u 1995]
RG304.5.U48084 1995
618.1′407543–dc20
DNLM/DLC.
for Library of Congress 94-37106
CIP

Published in the UK and Europe by
The Parthenon Publishing Group Limited
Casterton Hall, Carnforth
Lancs. LA6 2LA

Published in North America by
The Parthenon Publishing Group Inc.
One Blue Hill Plaza
Pearl River
New York 10965, USA

First published 1995

Composed by Servis Filmsetting Ltd, Longsight, Manchester
Printed and bound in Spain by T.G. Hostench, S.A.

Contents

List of principal contributors

F. Aleem
Department of Obstetrics and Gynecology
The Brookdale Hospital Medical Center
1335 Linden Boulevard
Brooklyn
New York 11212-3198
USA

M. Dietrich
Department of Obstetrics and Gynecology
University of Göttingen
Robert-Koch Str. 40
37075 Göttingen
Germany

Đ. Grbeša
Department of Histology and Embryology
School of Medicine
University of Zagreb
Salata 3
41000 Zagreb
Croatia

Lj. Kostović-Knežević
Department of Histology and Embryology
School of Medicine
University of Zagreb
Salata 3
41000 Zagreb
Croatia

D. Kulenkampff
Department of Obstetrics and Gynecology
University of Göttingen
Robert-Koch Str. 40
37075 Göttingen
Germany

S. Kupesic
Department of Obstetrics and Gynecology
University of Zagreb
Sveti Duh Hospital
Sveti Duh 64
Zagreb
Croatia

A. Kurjak
Department of Obstetrics and Gynecology
University of Zagreb
Sveti Duh Hospital
Sveti Duh 64
Zagreb
Croatia

R. Osmers
Department of Obstetrics and Gynecology
University of Göttingen
Robert-Koch Str. 40
37075 Göttingen
Germany

M. Predanic
The Brookdale Hospital Medical Center
1335 Linden Boulevard
Brooklyn
New York 11212-3198
USA

J. Puchta
Department of Obstetrics and Gynecology
University of Göttingen
Robert-Koch Str. 40
37075 Göttingen
Germany

A. Rempen
Department of Obstetrics and Gynecology
University of Würzburg
Josef-Schneider Str. 4
97080 Würzburg
Germany

A. Suren
Department of Obstetrics and Gynecology
University of Göttingen
Robert-Koch Str. 40
37075 Göttingen
Germany

COLOR PLATES

Color plate A Intramural leiomyoma. Color Doppler demonstrates a thick vessel (red and blue) encircling the leiomyoma at its anterior aspect

Color plate B Submucous leiomyoma surrounded by hyperechoic endometrium. Color Doppler demonstrates an increased vascularity at the base of the leiomyoma pedicle (arrowhead)

Color plate C Large leiomyoma, after laparoscopic electrocoagulation without the guidance of color Doppler. Note the high vascular density at the anterior aspect of the leiomyoma, indicating that coagulation missed the supplying blood vessels

Color plate D Uterine artery, detectable laterally to the cervix. Note the high velocity and high resistance to blood flow (resistance index = 0.92), typical of proliferative phase

Color plate E Blood flow velocity waveforms obtained from the uterine artery in the secretory phase show increased end-diastolic velocity and significantly lower blood flow impedance (resistance index = 0.81)

Color plate F Demonstration of the blood flow velocity waveforms obtained from the myometrium, representing radial artery blood flow (left). Note the lower impedance to blood flow (resistance index = 0.69) than observed in the main uterine artery (right)

Color plate G Flow velocity waveforms obtained from the homogeneous and hyperechoic endometrium represent spiral arteries (left). Note the lower velocity and lower resistance (resistance index = 0.49) than observed in the uterine arteries with larger diameter (left)

Color plate H Uterine artery: absent diastolic flow in the presence of a preovulatory follicle and normal estradiol levels in an infertile patient

Color plate I Posterior leiomyoma showing peripheral vascularization. Note that vascularization of this benign tumor is supported by normal existing (arcuate) arteries

Color plate J Transvaginal scan demonstrating submucous myoma with peripheral vascularization (left). Color signals explored by pulsed Doppler waveform analysis (right) shows moderate velocity and high-resistance blood flow. The benign nature of the tumor was confirmed by histopathology

Color plate K Posterior isoechoic leiomyoma showing regularly separated peripheral vessel (left). Waveform analysis (right) indicates high velocity (95.3 cm/s) and low resistance of the tumor blood flow (RI = 0.35). Necrosis, degenerative and inflammatory changes within the fibroid were confirmed by histopathology

Color plate L Color flow (left) indicates diffuse blood flow within the thickened, 'Swiss cheese' appearance of the myometrium in a patient suffering from endometriosis. Waveform analysis (right) shows moderate velocity and high-resistance (RI = 0.69) blood flow

Color plate M Transvaginal scan shows highly reflective echoes of intrauterine contraceptive device. Note increased vascularity of the endometrium and inner third of the myometrium in a patient suffering from pelvic inflammatory disease

Color plate N Short-axis view in a postmenopausal patient showing thickened endometrium measuring 13 mm. Note peripheral distribution of regularly separated vessels, typical of endometrial hyperplasia

Color plate O Oblique scan in a patient of reproductive age demonstrating a focal area of increased echogenicity (left). Waveform analysis (right) shows high-resistance blood flow (RI = 0.77) typical of endometrial polyp

Color plate P Transvaginal scan demonstrating cervical cystic structure (Nabothian cyst). Color Doppler signals extracted from its periphery demonstrate high impedance (RI = 0.78) to blood flow

Color plate Q Peripheral and intratumoral neovascularization in a case of endometrial carcinoma demonstrated by color Doppler (left). Doppler waveform analysis reveals low resistance index (RI = 0.43) (right)

Color plate R Randomly dispersed newly formed vessels in a case of uterine sarcoma. Note the inhomogenicity of the tumor produced by tumor degeneration, hemorrhage and presence of irregular vascular network (left). Pulsed Doppler analysis shows low resistance index (RI = 0.34) (right)

Color plate S Transvaginal color Doppler scan demonstrating cervical carcinoma. The anastomosing flow has a high systolic velocity of 42 cm/s and RI of 0.62

Color plate T Transvaginal scan (left) showing anechoic 'sausage like' structure that can easily be confused with a dilated tube. On the right, the same case is shown after color flow imaging. The anechoic area is formed by strongly dilated veins.

Color plate U Color Doppler demonstrating increased vascular congestion, and that vessels located in the uterine walls were also affected. This is the same patient as in Chapter 14, Figure 1

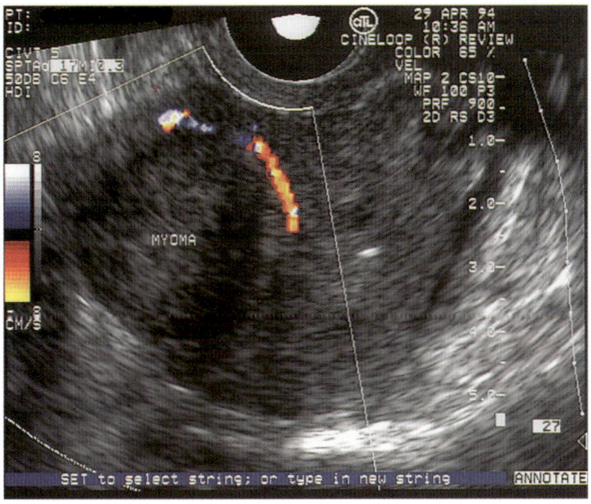
29 APR 94
10:36 AM
CINELOOP (R) REVIEW
MYOMA
SET to select string; or type in new string
ANNOTATE

A

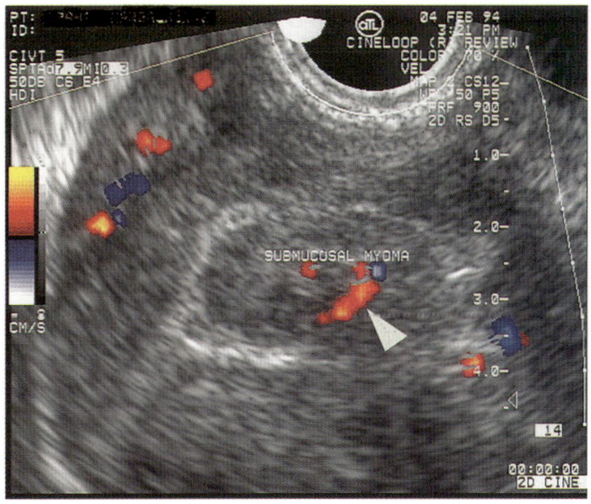
04 FEB 94
CINELOOP (R) REVIEW
SUBMUCOSAL MYOMA
2D CINE

B

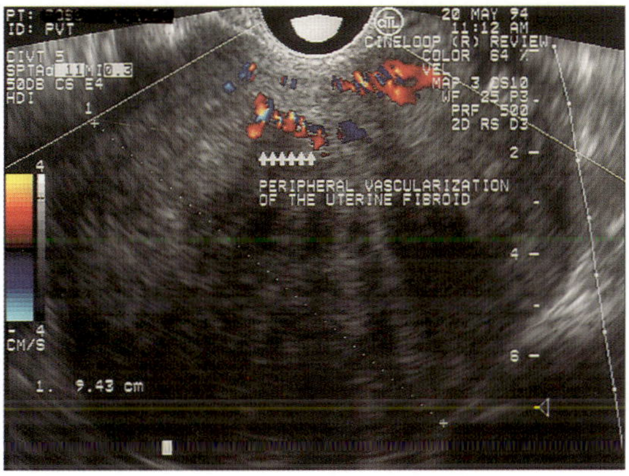
20 MAY 94
11:12 AM
CINELOOP (R) REVIEW
PERIPHERAL VASCULARIZATION
OF THE UTERINE FIBROID
1. 9.43 cm

C

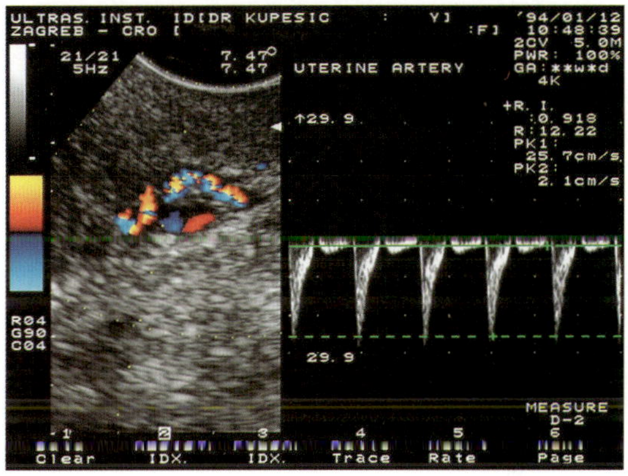
ULTRAS. INST. ID[DR KUPESIC
ZAGREB - CRO
'94/01/12
10:48:39
UTERINE ARTERY
MEASURE
D-2

D

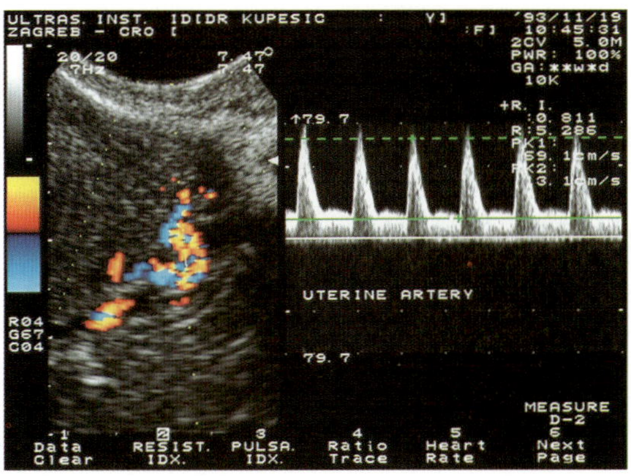
ULTRAS. INST. ID[DR KUPESIC
ZAGREB - CRO
'93/11/19
10:45:31
UTERINE ARTERY
MEASURE
D-2
Data Clear
RESIST. IDX.
PULSA. IDX.
Ratio Trace
Heart Rate
Next Page

E

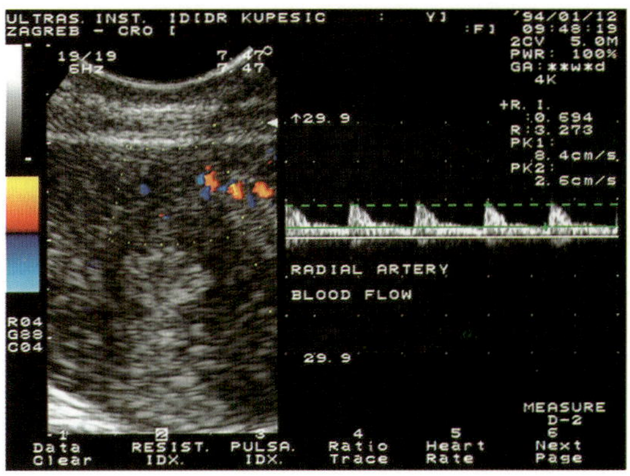
ULTRAS. INST. ID[DR KUPESIC
ZAGREB - CRO
'94/01/12
09:48:19
RADIAL ARTERY
BLOOD FLOW
MEASURE
D-2
Data Clear
RESIST. IDX.
PULSA. IDX.
Ratio Trace
Heart Rate
Next Page

F

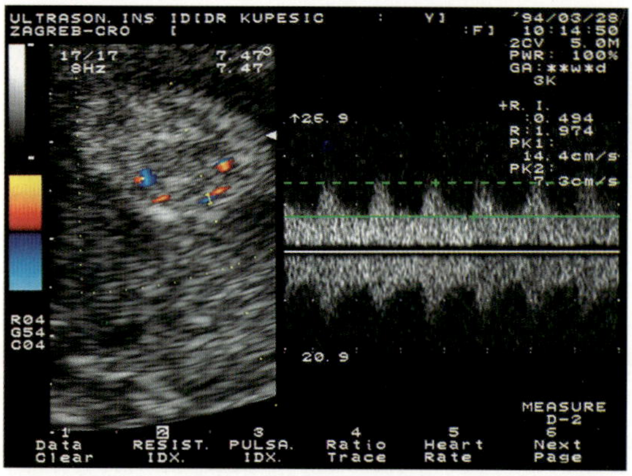
ULTRASON. INS ID[DR KUPESIC
ZAGREB-CRO
'94/03/28
MEASURE
Data Clear
RESIST. IDX.
PULSA. IDX.
Ratio Trace
Heart Rate
Next Page

G

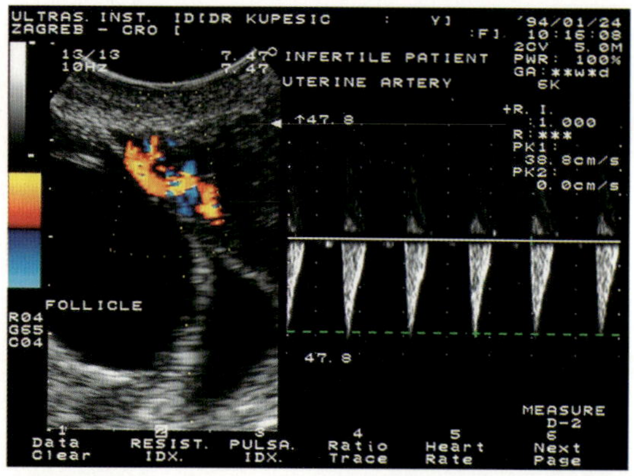
ULTRAS. INST. ID[DR KUPESIC
ZAGREB - CRO
'94/01/24
INFERTILE PATIENT
UTERINE ARTERY
FOLLICLE
MEASURE
Data Clear
RESIST. IDX.
PULSA. IDX.
Ratio Trace
Heart Rate
Next Page

H

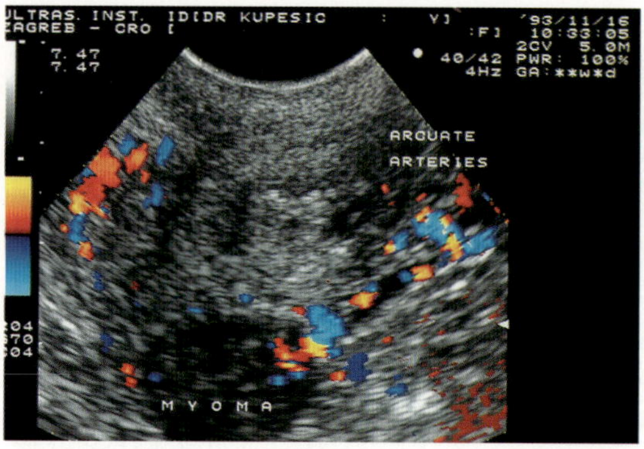
ULTRAS. INST. ID[DR KUPESIC
ZAGREB - CRO
'93/11/16
ARCUATE
ARTERIES
M Y O M A

I

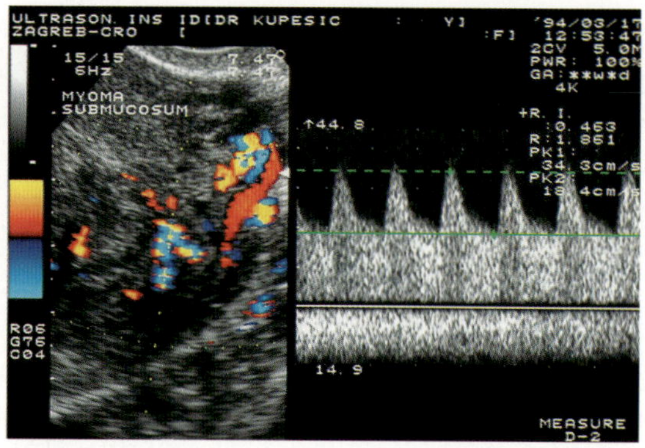
ULTRASON. INS ID[DR KUPESIC
ZAGREB-CRO
'94/03/17
MYOMA
SUBMUCOSUM
MEASURE

J

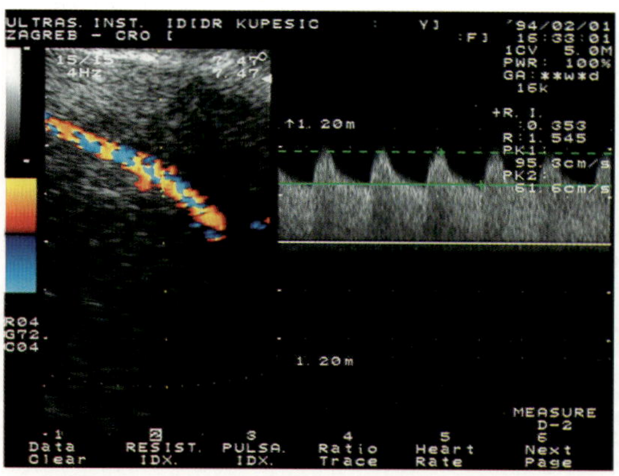
ULTRAS. INST. ID[DR KUPESIC
ZAGREB - CRO
'94/02/01
MEASURE
Data Clear
RESIST. IDX.
PULSA. IDX.
Ratio Trace
Heart Rate
Next Page

K

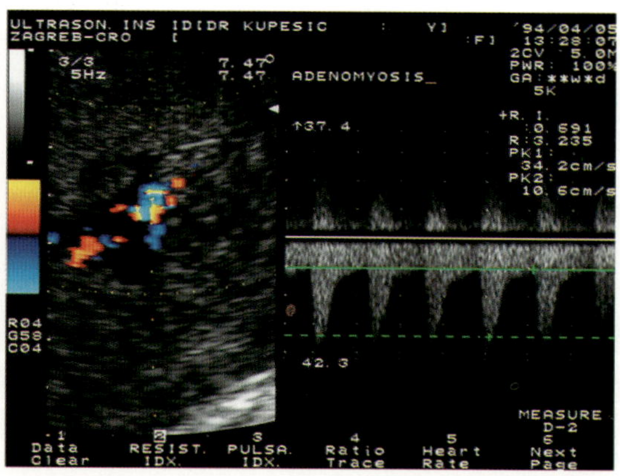
ULTRASON. INS ID[DR KUPESIC
ZAGREB-CRO
'94/04/05
ADENOMYOSIS_
MEASURE
Data Clear
RESIST. IDX.
PULSA. IDX.
Ratio Trace
Heart Rate
Next Page

L

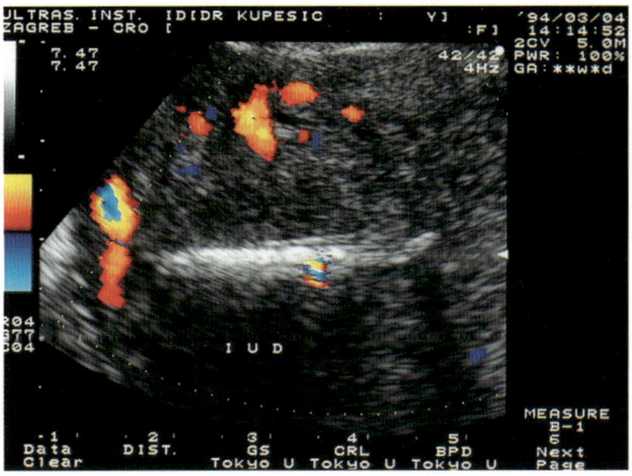
ULTRAS. INST. ID:DR KUPESIC
ZAGREB - CRO
'94/03/04
14:14:52
I U D
MEASURE
B-1
Data Clear
DIST.
GS
CRL
BPD
Next Page

M

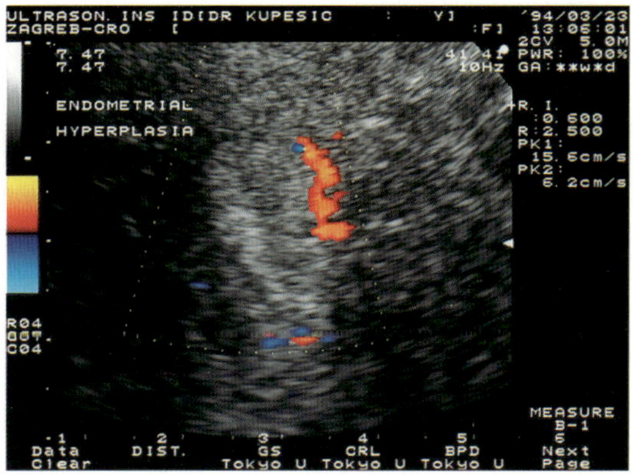
ULTRASON. INS ID:DR KUPESIC
ZAGREB-CRO
'94/03/23
13:06:01
ENDOMETRIAL
HYPERPLASIA
R. I.
:0. 600
R:2. 500
PK1:
15. 6cm/s
PK2:
6. 2cm/s
MEASURE
B-1
Data Clear
DIST.
GS
CRL
BPD
Next Page

N

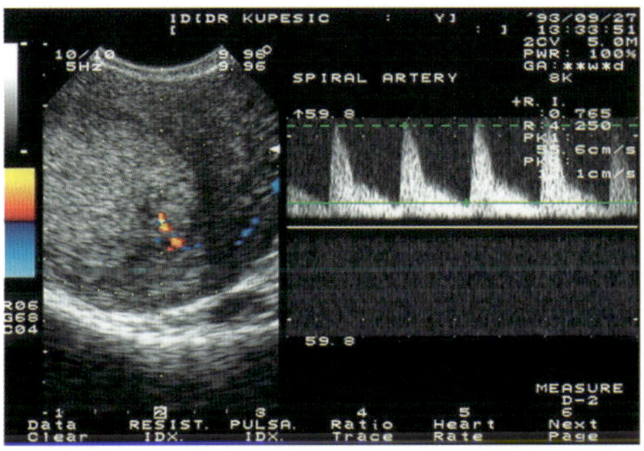
ID:DR KUPESIC
'93/09/27
13:33:51
SPIRAL ARTERY
R. I.
:0. 765
R:4. 250
59. 8
MEASURE
D-2
Data Clear
RESIST. IDX.
PULSA. IDX.
Ratio Trace
Heart Rate
Next Page

O

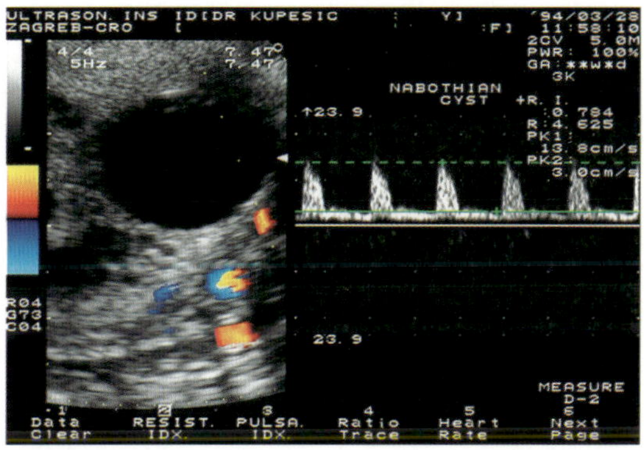
ULTRASON. INS ID:DR KUPESIC
ZAGREB-CRO
'94/03/28
11:58:10
NABOTHIAN
CYST
R. I.
:0. 784
R:4. 625
PK1:
13. 8cm/s
PK2:
3. 0cm/s
23. 9
MEASURE
D-2
Data Clear
RESIST. IDX.
PULSA. IDX.
Ratio Trace
Heart Rate
Next Page

P

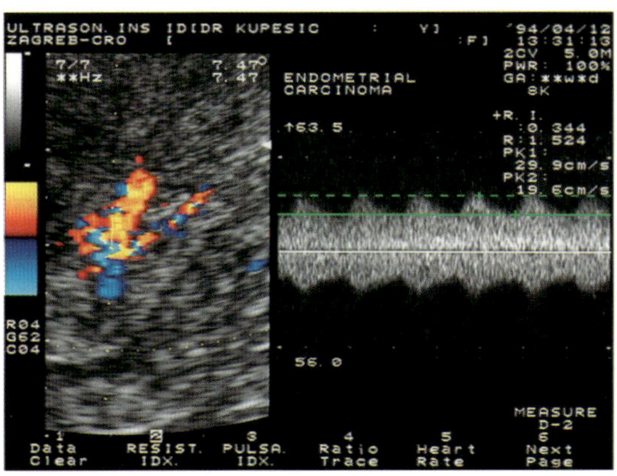
ULTRASON. INS ID:DR KUPESIC
ZAGREB-CRO
'94/04/12
13:31:13
ENDOMETRIAL
CARCINOMA
R. I.
:0. 344
R:1. 524
PK1:
29. 9cm/s
PK2:
19. 6cm/s
63. 5
56. 0
MEASURE
D-2
Data Clear
RESIST. IDX.
PULSA. IDX.
Ratio Trace
Heart Rate
Next Page

Q

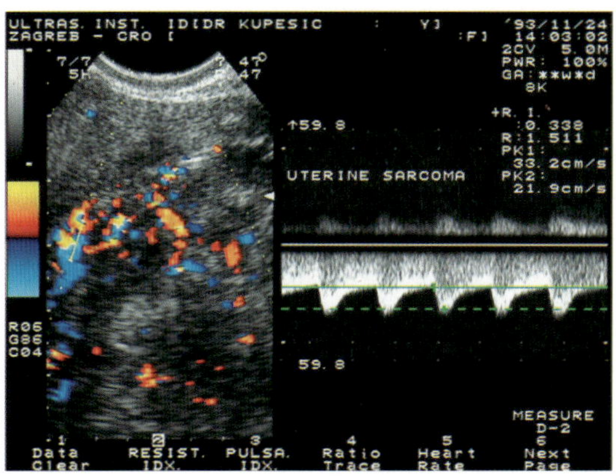
ULTRAS. INST. ID:DR KUPESIC
ZAGREB - CRO
'93/11/24
14:03:02
UTERINE SARCOMA
R. I.
:0. 338
R:1. 511
PK1:
33. 2cm/s
PK2:
21. 9cm/s
59. 8
MEASURE
D-2
Data Clear
RESIST. IDX.
PULSA. IDX.
Ratio Trace
Heart Rate
Next Page

R

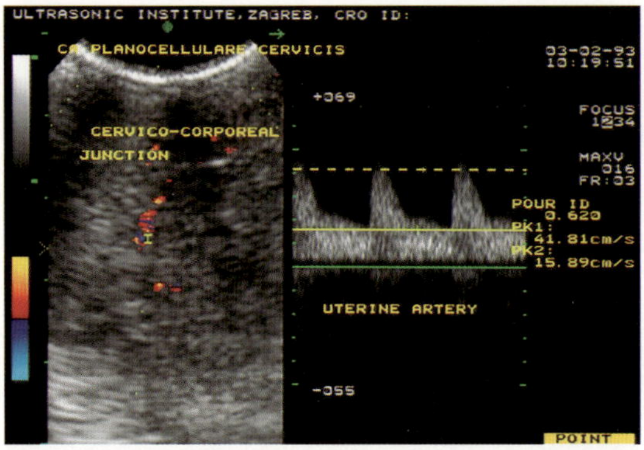
ULTRASONIC INSTITUTE, ZAGREB, CRO ID:
CA PLANOCELLULARE CERVICIS
03-02-93
10:19:51
+069
FOCUS
CERVICO-CORPOREAL
JUNCTION
MAXV
016
FR:03
POUR ID
0.620
PK1:
41.81cm/s
PK2:
15.89cm/s
UTERINE ARTERY
-055
POINT

S

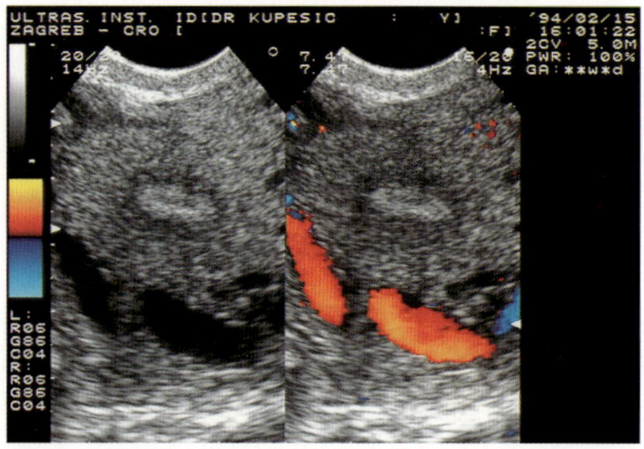
ULTRAS. INST. ID[DR KUPESIC : Y]
ZAGREB - CRO [:F]
'94/02/15
16:01:22
2CV 5.0M
PWR: 100%
GA:**w*d

T

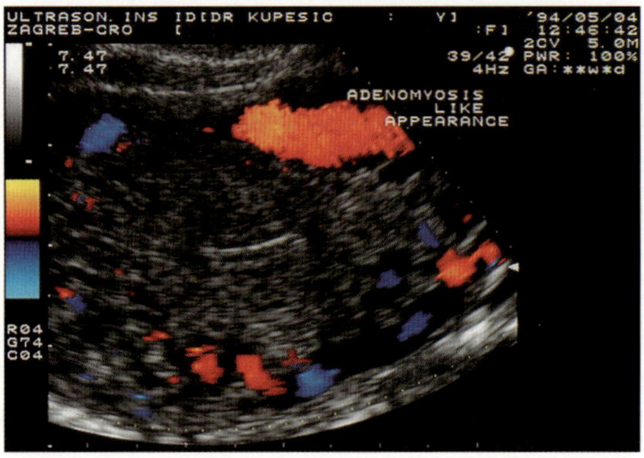
ULTRASON. INS ID[DR KUPESIC : Y]
ZAGREB-CRO [:F]
'94/05/04
12:46:42
2CV 5.0M
7.47
7.47
39/42 PWR: 100%
4Hz GA:**w*d
ADENOMYOSIS
LIKE
APPEARANCE
R04
G74
C04

U

Progress in Obstetric and Gynecological Sonography Series

An ongoing series documenting recent advances in key subject areas, with a new volume scheduled for publication approximately every 3 months.

Titles currently planned in the Series include:

Ultrasound and the Ovary	A. Kurjak (Croatia)
Ultrasound and the Fetal Brain	F. A. Chervenak (USA), A. Kurjak (Croatia) and C. Comstock (USA)
Ultrasound and the Uterus	A. Kurjak (Croatia) and R. Osmers (Germany)
Ultrasound and Early Pregnancy	D. Jurković (UK) and E. Jauniaux (UK)
Ultrasound and the Fallopian Tubes	I. E. Timor-Tritsch (USA) and A. Kurjak (Croatia)
Ultrasound and Fetal Heart	J. W. Wladimiroff (The Netherlands) and G. Pilu (Italy)
Ultrasound and Fetal Growth	J. M. Carrera (Spain), K. Maeda (Japan) and G. P. Mandruzzato (Italy)
Three-dimensional Ultrasound	K. Baba (Japan) and D. Jurković (UK)
Ultrasound and Infertility	A. Kurjak (Croatia) and W. Feichtinger (Austria)
Ultrasound and Endoscopic Surgery	S. Kupešić (Croatia) and M. Goldenberg (Israel)
Ultrasound and Prenatal Diagnosis	W. Holzgreve (Germany) and D. A. Nyberg (USA)
Doppler in Gynecology	A. Kurjak (Croatia) and H. Shulman (USA)
Doppler in Obstetrics	K. Maršál (Sweden) and B. J. Trudinger (Australia)
Safety of Diagnostic Ultrasound	G. Kossoff (Australia) and S. Barnett (Australia)
Ultrasound and Fetal Therapy	C. Rodeck (UK) and M. Evans (USA)

From an exciting novelty, ultrasound has now become the best single diagnostic technique available in obstetrics and gynecology. The original excitement is, of course, still felt by many of us. One cannot stop wondering how many applications of this relatively simple invention the future will hold. On the other hand, the wave of interest created by the present possibilities is spreading rapidly through almost all major journals. Any interested individual will find it difficult to read or even scan all of these articles, although he might wish to do so. The purpose of this newly conceived series of books is to overcome the problem by providing expert, up-to-date analyses of current advances in each specialized topic.

This new series is dedicated to the in-depth evaluation of the latest developments and advances in an area where progress is on a wide front and where diagnostic potential changes so rapidly. Each book contains critical reviews by leading experts, backed up by the best bibliographical information available. Unique and contemporary in concept, design and content, the new series provides a timely and continuing resource of expert information in a highly readable, consistent format.

It is hoped that this unique series will promote current awareness and help clinicians and research workers to keep abreast of today's most significant research and current developments.

Therefore titles in this series will be produced accurately, concisely and rapidly over a short time period. The chapters provide not only essential new data, but also serve as guides for interpretation of the literature and to the repercussions for clinical practice. In other words, the objective of each book is to inform our colleagues of the evidence and data available on the topic concerned, how reliable this information appears to be and what conclusions may be drawn from it. It should be a tool for distinguishing facts from fiction.

We believe that these new volumes will prove to be major sources of innovative ideas and effective solutions for the practice of obstetric and gynecological sonography.

Asim Kurjak
Series Editor

Normal sonographic features of the uterus

1

A. Rempen

The uterus is situated above the vagina in the small pelvis. Its anterior wall lies next to the bladder, its posterior wall next to the rectum. Normally, the uterus is anteverted and anteflexed, retroflexion being a normal clinical feature. Due to its mobility, the uterus can be inclined from the median position to the lateral or can be rotated around its longitudinal axis.

The uterus is a pear-shaped organ. It can be divided into the portio, the cervix and the corpus with the fundus uteri. It consists mainly of smooth muscles (myometrium). The uterine cavity and the cervical canal are covered by mucosa, the endometrium. The part of the uterus lying intraperitoneally is covered by a thin smooth layer of serosa, the peritoneum. Individual differences in size are considerable, the size of the organ changing independently of an existing pregnancy or disease during a woman's lifetime. The uterus undergoes hormonal influences, becoming noticeable in the sonographic picture mainly because of variability of uterine size and the structure of the endometrium.

Before sonographic examination is undertaken, gynecological inspection and palpation are recommended, as the conjunction of ultrasound and clinical findings is the best guarantee that the correct diagnosis will be made. Bimanual examination gives a first impression of uterine size and position, and thus facilitates the guiding of the probe.

If transabdominal sonography of the uterus is performed, a filled urinary bladder acting as a physiological acoustic window is an indispensable condition, because otherwise the organ will be overlayed by intestinal loops filled with air, that cannot be traversed by ultrasound waves. This is in particular true for retroflexion of the uterus, but a steeply anteflexed uterus cannot be judged sufficiently either – even when it is close to the abdominal wall, as the ultrasound waves penetrate the organ tangentially, making it difficult to visualize exactly the borderline between endometrium and myometrium, due to the lack of reflections.

In transvaginal sonography, the probe is placed nearer to the organ, due to its localization in the anterior, posterior or lateral vaginal vault, and the patient does not therefore need to fill the urinary bladder. As a result of increased proximity to the uterus, higher-frequency transducers can be used, and thus images of higher resolution can be obtained. A stretched uterus in an older woman can cause problems as far as imaging of the corpus is concerned; this is due to the tangential course of the ultrasonic waves.

Comparative examinations of transabdominal and transvaginal sonography confirmed the superiority of the vaginal technique in 60–85% of cases, with the transabdominal approach being more favorable in 3–5%[1,2]. In 10–36% there was no difference in the quality of the pictures.

Regardless of whether transabdominal or transvaginal sonography is performed, it has proved to be useful to check the small pelvis in longitudinal sections first. After this, viewing of the lower abdomen in the transverse plane (transabdominal technique) or in the frontal plane (transvaginal technique) follows. This gives an estimate of the variable position of the uterus. The uterus is then scanned in longitudinal sections from one side to the other. The echogenic endometrium is a reliable guideline in the search for the uterine longitudinal axis. Viewing of the uterus in cross-sections from the fundus to the cervix then follows.

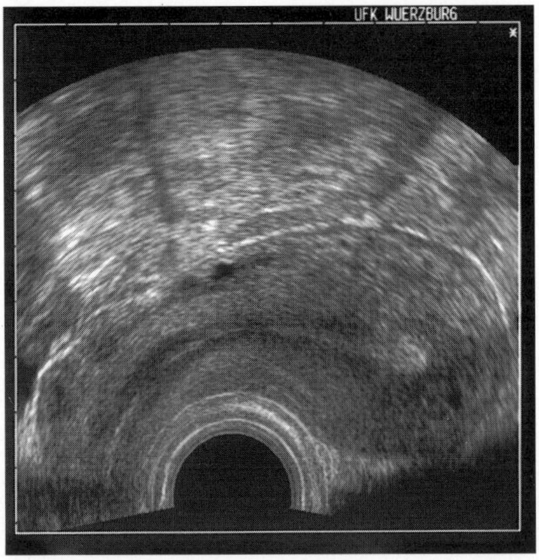

Figure 1 Anteflexed uterus in longitudinal section (right, fundus; left, cervix); endometrium and cervical canal echogenic, submucous myometrium hypoechogenic; echoless vessel structures in the periphery

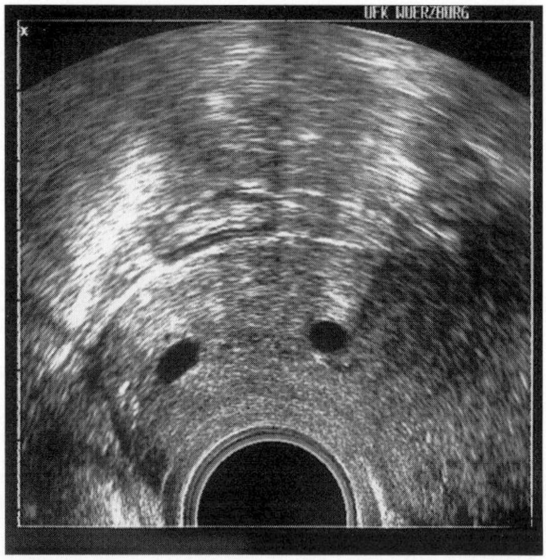

Figure 2 Cervix in longitudinal section (overframing: the corpus uteri is partly cut in the right margin of the picture); ovulum Nabothi of the portio (left); dilated cervical gland appears cystic (right)

BIOMETRY OF THE UTERUS

In the longitudinal plane, the corpus and cervix of the uterus are shaped like a pear. On sonograms, the uterus can be divided into three sections, corresponding to three reflection patterns. The endometrium usually images as a bright structure, whereas the myometrium has a moderate level of echogenicity (Figure 1). The endometrium is surrounded by a small hyporeflective line, related to the inner muscle layers[3]. This dark line does not alter its thickness during the menstrual cycle.

Imaging of the cervix is often more difficult than imaging of the corpus. This is a result of ultrasonic wave artefacts, which are due to the direct proximity of the probe to the cervix. It might be necessary to draw the probe back a little into the vagina, and thus enable the cervix to move into the focal region. The cervix, measuring about 4 cm, should be examined first in the longitudinal plane. This enables the cervical canal to be distinguished. If it is distended – in particular around the mid-cycle – by cervical mucus, it has a low-level echotexture. During the secretory phase, however, it appears echogenic. Naboth's ovules may appear like holes punched into the cervix (Figure 2). Cystic structures along the cervical canal correspond to dilated cervical glands.

Childhood

Examination of the uterus in a child can be performed either transabdominally with a full bladder, or perineally. The uterus in the newborn is relatively large, having a volume of 6 cm^3 (Table 1). The endometrium often appears as a bright line, surrounded by a hypoechogenic band of inner layer of myometrium[4,5]. This echo texture and the size of the uterus are said to be due to the effect of prenatal estrogen. In the neonatal period the cervix predominates over the corpus (Table 2), the cervix at times measuring twice the size of the corpus. In the course of the 1st year of life the uterus involutes to one-third of the volume of that in the newborn (Figure 3). Until the age of 7–10 years, an endocrine rest period follows, with no significant change of uterine size[5,6], which is about 3 cm in length, and about 1.5 cm^3 in volume (Figure 4). The endometrium often cannot be delimited in this period of life. The corpus–cervix ratio is 1:1. Between the 7th and 10th year of life, the uterus starts to grow continuously. After slow growth of length in the beginning, rapid growth of

Table 1 Measurements of the uterus (mean ± SD) by age (from reference 5)

Age	*n*	*Longitudinal diameter* (mm)	*Anterior–posterior diameter* (mm)	*Transverse diameter* (mm)	*Volume* (cm³)	*Corpus : cervix ratio (longitudinal diameter)*
Week 1–4	26	44 ± 6	15 ± 3	18 ± 3	6.6 ± 2.9	1:2.3(0.4 ± 0.1)
Month 2–12	24	26 ± 6	9 ± 2	12 ± 4	1.6 ± 0.9	1:1.2(0.8 ± 0.1)
Year 1–3	21	27 ± 5	7 ± 2	11 ± 2	1.2 ± 0.5	1:1.1(0.9 ± 0.2)
Year 4–6	25	28 ± 6	8 ± 2	14 ± 3	1.8 ± 0.9	1:1.0(1.0 ± 0.2)
Year 7–8	33	32 ± 6	8 ± 2	14 ± 3	2.1 ± 1.2	1:0.8(1.3 ± 0.3)
Year 9–10	27	36 ± 8	12 ± 4	19 ± 5	4.8 ± 3.5	1:0.8(1.3 ± 0.3)
Year 11–12	23	49 ± 15	18 ± 9	28 ± 10	18.6 ± 18.2	1:0.6(1.6 ± 0.4)
Year 13–14	34	61 ± 10	23 ± 6	32 ± 8	24.3 ± 13.2	1:0.6(1.8 ± 0.4)
Year 15–16	17	66 ± 10	24 ± 4	32 ± 5	26.7 ± 8.3	1:0.6(1.7 ± 0.3)

Table 2 Diameter and volume of cervix and corpus uteri (mean ± SD) in the neonate ($n = 41$) (from reference 4)

Uterine measures	*Cervix*	*Corpus*	*p value*
Longitudinal diameter (mm)	21.5 ± 3.4	18.6 ± 3.4	< 0.01
Anterior–posterior diameter (mm)	17.1 ± 2.7	10.6 ± 2.2	< 0.001
Transverse diameter (mm)	18.4 ± 3.0	11.4 ± 1.6	< 0.001
Volume (cm³)	3.65 ± 1.36	1.18 ± 0.42	< 0.001

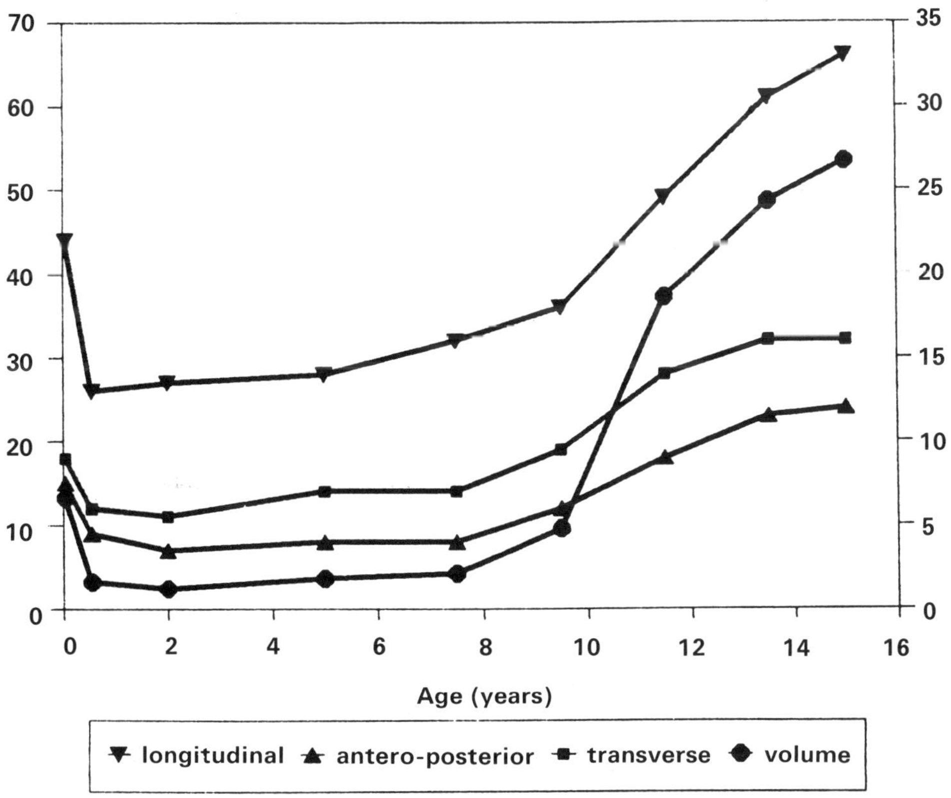

Figure 3 Growth of uterus: diameter and calculated volume with age (mean values, $n = 230$) (from reference 5)

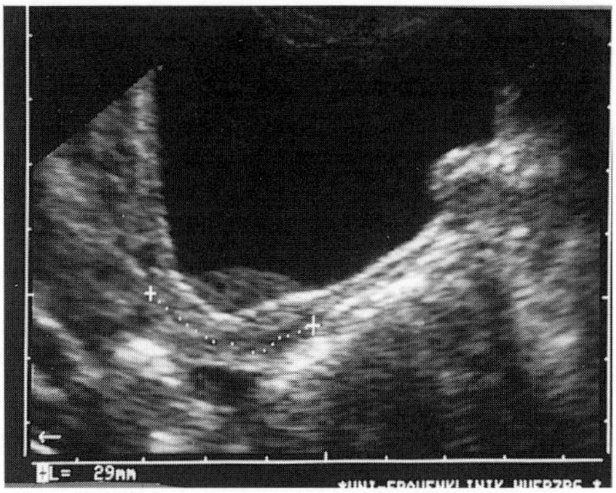

Figure 4 Transabdominal scan of the longitudinal section of the uterus (+) in a child. Corpus (left) and cervix (right) have the same size

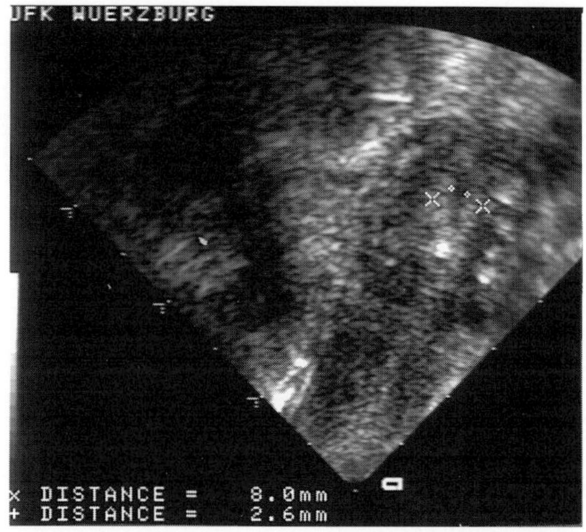

Figure 5 Stretched uterus in the postmenopause (longitudinal section) with peripheral zones of arteriosclerosis. The tangential section makes the delimitation of the endometrium appear unclear. The measured diameter of the endometrium includes the slightly dilated uterine cavity

volume can be observed, in particular of the corpus, which has increased 20-fold by the time of menarche. With the beginning of menarche, the uterus shows the adult pear shape. The ratio of the length of the corpus to the cervix is 2:1.

Pre- and postmenopause

The corpus is about 5–7 cm long. The uterine wall is smooth and clearly outlined against its surroundings (Figure 1). In the myometrium, towards its periphery and often protruding, can be found echoless vessels. In the postmenopause the arteries can calcify in this region. These calcifications appear as small, bright reflections, regularly spread in the uterine wall (Figure 5). They can evoke shadowing, which may impair the assessment of structures lying beyond, e.g. the endometrium.

In the uterine transverse section the fundal evulsions of the mucosa, directed towards the tubal ostium, can be seen (Figure 6).

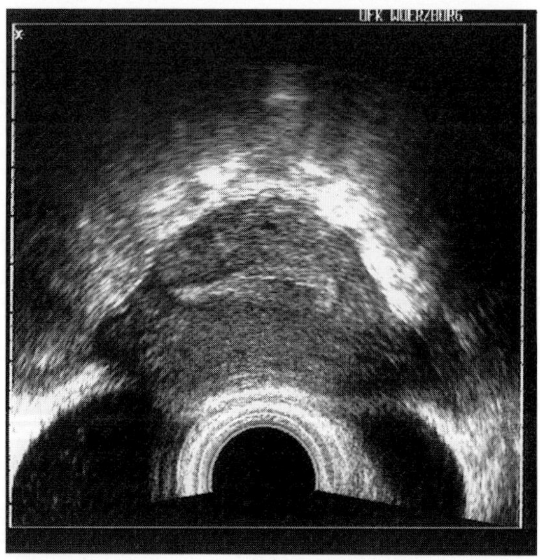

Figure 6 Oblique transverse section through the fundus uteri: peaked evulsion of the endometrium near the right tubal exit (on the left side of the picture)

Corresponding to the intrauterine pressure waves, known from catheter measurements[7], uterine contractions can be seen with transvaginal sonography, in all phases of the cycle[8]. These undulatory motions occur around the time of menstruation with a frequency of approximately 2.3 contractions/min (range 0.5–6/min) and are directed towards the internal mouth of the womb. During the other phases of the cycle, the frequency is on average 3.3/min (range 0.5–9/min), in a retrograde direction towards the fundus. The frequency of the contraction waves is highest and the covered distance is greatest around the time of ovulation.

Of the uterine fixing ligaments, the broad and round ligaments can be visualized sonographically, only if there is sufficient abdominal fluid in the small pelvis. Paracervical uterine vessels appear sonographically as multiple 'cystic' areas on both sides of the cervical canal. They must not be confounded with the ovaries or space-occupying lesions.

Whereas palpation provides only a subjective estimation of uterine size, sonography allows exact measurement of the uterus and its different parts, e.g. thickness of the endometrium. Follow-up measurements allow objective recording of changes. For determination of uterine size, three planes, perpendicular to one another, are considered[9]. The longitudinal and anterior–posterior diameters are checked in the uterine longitudinal plane; the transverse diameter in the uterine transverse plane. The longitudinal diameter extends from the highest fundal point in the midline to the portio. Under transabdominal sonography, the uterus is stretched as a result of the filled bladder, and therefore the longitudinal diameter can be read directly, but under transvaginal sonography, with an emptied bladder, flexion of the uterus has to be compensated for, in order to avoid measurements that are too short. This can be achieved either by separately measuring the straight distances fundus–isthmus and isthmus–portio and adding them together afterwards, or by travelling along the curved distance with the cursor in the uterine midline, provided this is possible with the sonograph that is used (Figure 7). The anterior–posterior diameter corresponds to the largest distance between the anterior and posterior wall; the uterine transverse diameter coincides with the largest distance of the uterine lateral walls in the corpus section. The lateral boundaries of the uterus are sometimes difficult to determine, due to the broad ligaments departing from this region. Comparative measurements in samples of uteri with a tape-measure showed a good correspondence with preoperative transabdominal ultrasound biometry[10].

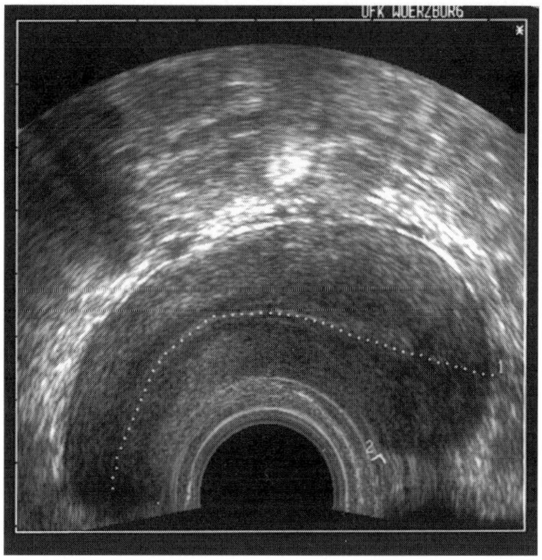

Figure 7 Vaginosonographic longitudinal section of the uterus: bow-shaped longitudinal diameter of the uterus (C1) (83 mm) and anterior–posterior diameter (D2) (34 mm)

The womb is smaller in nulliparous women than in women who have given birth[9,11] (Tables 3 and 4, Figures 8 and 9). From this, it follows that uterine weight depends on parity. Antecedent abortions or therapy with sexual steroids, however, are of no influence. For clinical practice upper standard values of 80 × 40 × 50 mm (longitudinal × anterior–posterior × transverse) in the premenopause have proved to be worthwhile. Higher values are not automatically pathological, but should give rise to a thorough search for the possible cause. They should suggest myoma, adenomyosis, uterine malformations, a pregnancy or erroneous inclusion of an ovary in the measurement.

Table 3 Uterine diameter (mean ± SD) with regard to parity and menopausal status ($n = 137$) (from reference 11)

	Premenopause		
Uterine measures	*Nullipara* ($n = 9$)	*Para* ($n = 52$)	*Postmenopause* ($n = 76$)
Longitudinal diameter (mm)	71 ± 8	89 ± 10	79 ± 12
Anterior–posterior diameter (mm)	46 ± 6	58 ± 8	49 ± 8
Transverse diameter (mm)	33 ± 8	43 ± 6	32 ± 7

Table 4 Uterine measures (median and 5–95 centiles) by age (from reference 9)

Age (years)	*n*	*Longitudinal diameter* (mm)	*Anterior–posterior diameter* (mm)	*Transverse diameter* (mm)	*Estimated weight* (g)
Nullipara ($n = 385$)					
15–19	18	69.5	32	44	60
20–29	137	72 (57.2–89)	34 (26.2–43.9)	45 (36–58.9)	66 (44–101.9)
30–39	100	76 (60.3–90)	37 (27–47)	47 (38.3–59)	75 (51–116.8)
40–49	61	76 (58–93)	36.5 (22.5–46.8)	47.5 (33.3–64)	75 (42.3–126.8)
50–59	34	60.5 (43.8–81.3)	30.5 (21.5–44.3)	40.5 (29.8–54.5)	52 (37–93.8)
60–69	15	56	24	35.5	41
⩾70	20	47 (30.5–69.5)	20 (13.2–37.3)	29 (21–44.7)	34.5 (28.2–61.7)
Para ($n = 452$)					
20–29	47	80 (61.2–96.4)	41 (28.4–56.8)	53 (38.2–69)	84 (50.6–144.2)
30–39	125	81 (64.3–100.7)	42 (32.3–53)	51 (38.9–65.7)	92 (59.6–151)
40–49	117	81 (64.0–100.0)	43 (30–54)	52.5 (38.2–66)	93 (53–146.9)
50–59	70	68 (46.6–94.9)	35 (22–49.4)	46 (34–62.5)	66.5 (38–127.5)
60–69	40	55 (36.3–70.2)	26 (16.3–35.7)	39 (22.3–46)	45 (30.3–63.7)
⩾70	53	53 (38.5–74.5)	25 (19–40.5)	37.5 (25.8–48.5)	41.5 (32.8–71.8)

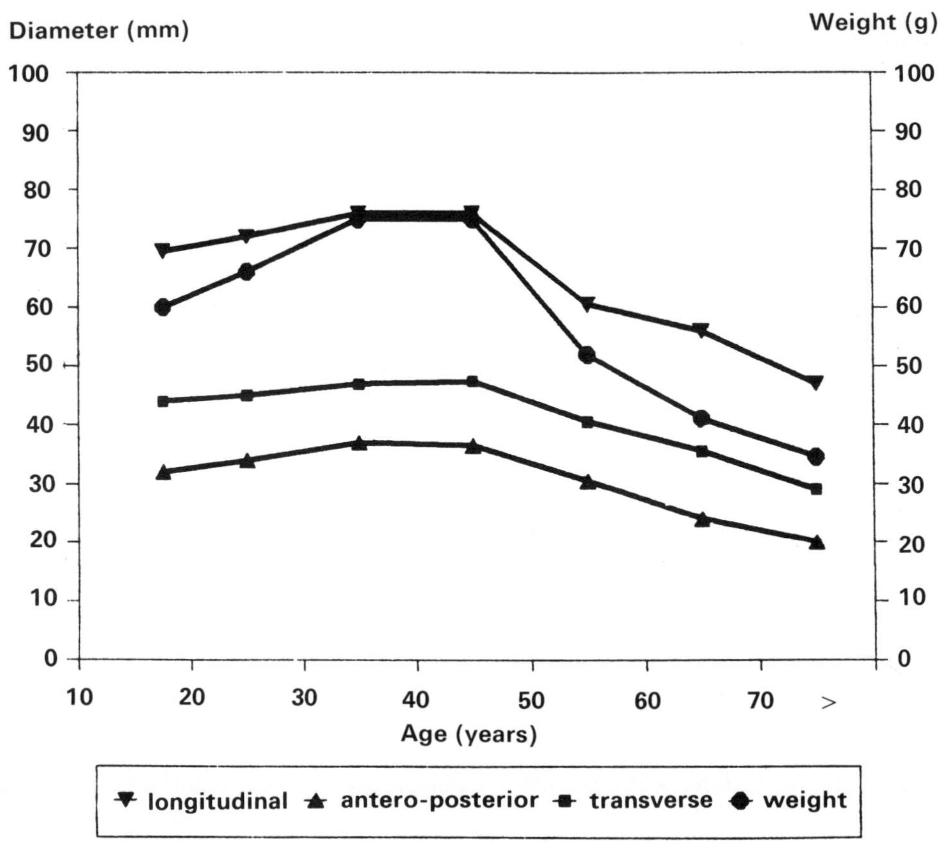

Figure 8 Diameter of uterus and estimated weight against age in women who had not given birth (50th centile, $n = 385$) Diamonds, longitudinal diameter; squares, transverse diameter; triangles, anterior–posterior diameter, circles, weight (from reference 9)

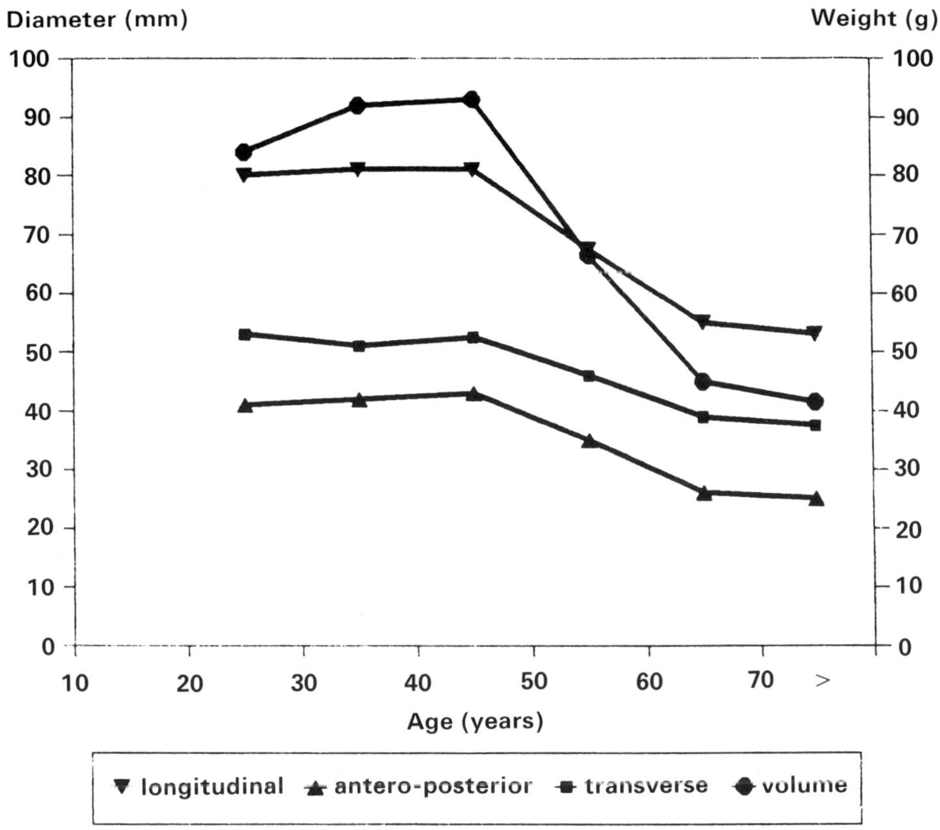

Figure 9 Diameter of uterus and estimated weight against age in women who had given birth (50th centile, $n=454$) Diamonds, longitudinal diameter; squares, transverse diameter; triangles, anterior–posterior diameter; circles, weight (from reference 9)

In the postmenopause, the possibility is uterine involution. In screening examinations, the mean length of the postmenopausal uterus was shown to be 59 ± 11 mm (range 35–97 mm)[12].

Uterine volume can be determined adequately by use of the ellipsoid formula: length × depth × breadth × 0.5233. Uterine weight can be deduced from the volume, one milliliter equalling one gram[11]. Evaluation of the weight of the uterus from its dimensions by means of linear regression analysis shows that true weight is within a range of −32 to +47% of the estimated weight[9].

SONOMORPHOLOGICAL CHANGES OF THE ENDOMETRIUM

The hormone-dependent endometrium shows a different appearance in the premenopause, depending on female age and phase of the menstrual cycle. In the uterine sagittal section, the two mucosa layers of the anterior and posterior wall, lying on top of each other, are to be seen. Between these two layers, the uterine cavity can often be imaged as an echogenic stripe. If there is some fluid in the cavity, this leads to distension, presenting itself as an echoless area. The borderline between the endometrium and the more hypoechogenic myometrium is smooth and clearly contoured.

When reviewing the references on the thickness of the endometrium, it should be taken into account whether one or both endometrium layers have been included in the measurement. As it is not possible – in particular in the postmenopause – to separate the two endometrium layers sonographically, it has proved useful to take both mucosa layers together in the anterior–posterior diameter and to refer to this as the twofold endometrial thickness (Figure 10). The sagittal

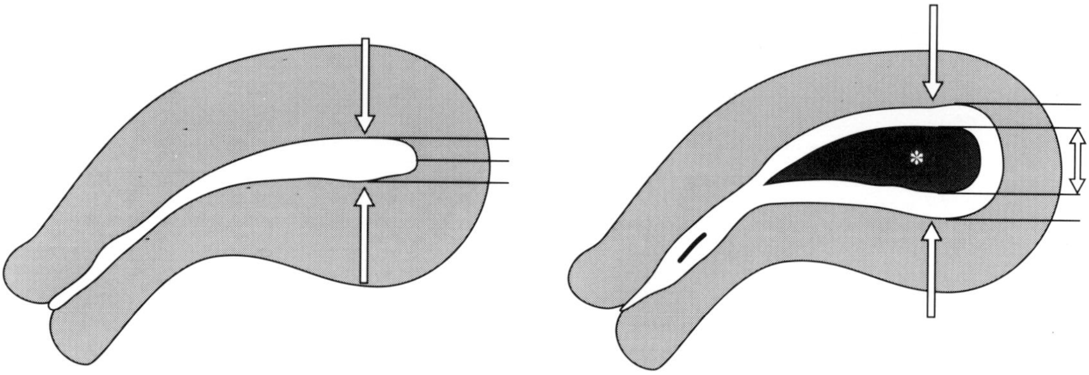

Figure 10 Determination of (double) thickness of the endometrium. Left, with a cavity that is not visible; right, with a serometra (asterisk), the diameter of which (small arrows) is deducted from the total diameter (large arrows)

diameter of a possible serometra has to be subtracted from this value. Transabdominal measurements of endometrial thickness have corresponded well both with *in vitro* measurements and with data found in pathological examinations[13].

The endometrium in premenopausal women

In the regenerative phase of life, the endometrium is subject to cyclic hormonal influences and changes. These are reflected in its different tissue states and its sonographic appearances. In transabdominal studies, good correspondence has been shown between sonographic findings and histologically determined menstrual phase by means of endometrial biopsies[14]. The sonographic pattern and growth of the endometrium in the normal cycle have also been examined in transvaginal studies[15–17].

In the first week of the menstrual cycle, the endometrium appears as a thin linear echo. In the beginning of the second week, the inner part of the endometrium is hypoechogenic, with the contact area of the two endometrium layers lying on top of each other imaging as a hyper-reflective line. The borderline between the endometrium and the hypoechogenic myometrium presents itself as a bright band (Figure 11). The hypoechogenic endometrium layer is possibly the result of edema. Both endometrium layers together now measure 7 mm.

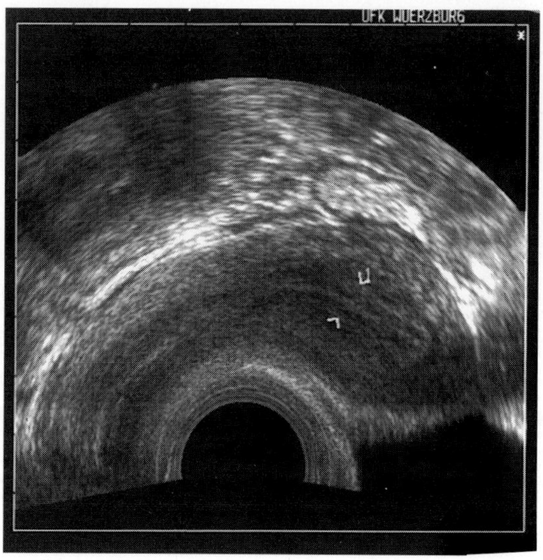

Figure 11 Endometrium on the 7th day of the cycle. Poor echogenicity of the inner layers (diameter, D1 = 7 mm)

In the following days, the thickness of the hypodense endometrium layers increases in correlation with the rise of estradiol (Table 5). Growth of the endometrium does not differ very greatly between hormonally stimulated cycles and spontaneous cycles[15,18]. By the time of ovulation, the inner hypoechogenic zones have achieved their maximal thickness, causing the three hyperechogenic lines to become more evident (Figure 12). In the uterine transverse section, the structure of the endometrium resembles the Greek letter theta (θ)[16]. The anterior–posterior diameter of both endometrium layers now averages 12 mm.

Table 5 Thickness of the endometrium and serum estradiol levels (mean and range) in the proliferative stage ($n=22$) (modified from reference 17)

Day of the cycle	*n*	*Thickness of the endometrium* (mm)	*Estradiol level* (pmol/l)
1–5	17	4.6 (2.5–6.0)	139 (50–200)
6–7	3	5.3 (3.6–6.2)	174 (114–290)
8–9	7	7.1 (5.6–9.1)	258 (152–360)
9	7	9.2 (5.0–11.4)	280 (220–450)
11	12	9.4 (7.5–12.0)	395 (270–650)
12	14	10.9 (7.7–13.4)	616 (230–1290)
13	20	11.2 (8.2 15.0)	876 (430 1450)
14	16	12.4 (10.0–15.9)	970 (320–1710)

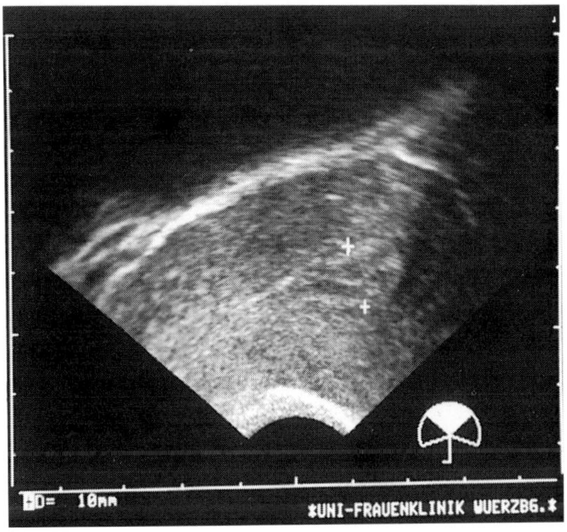

Figure 12 Endometrium at the time of ovulation. Cavity line and basal endometrium layers appear protrusive through the hyporeflective proliferated mucosa (diameter, D = 10 mm)

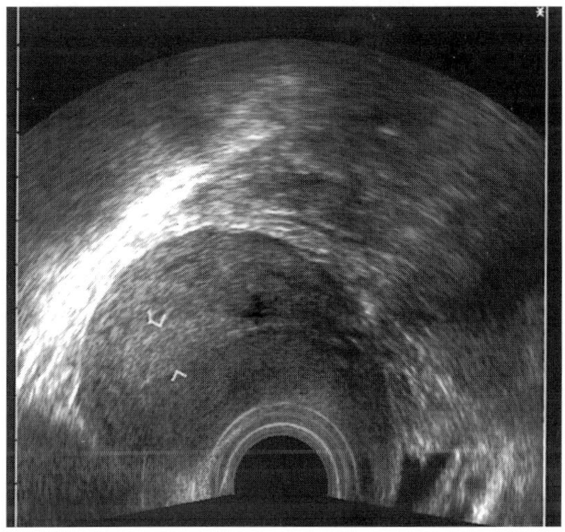

Figure 13 Endometrium on day 20 of the cycle. As a result of the homogeneous echogenicity, the endometrium cavity could not be delimited. Retroflexion of the uterus (diameter, D1 = 11 mm)

During the first week after ovulation, echogenicity continues to increase – first in the basal parts, then also in the upper parts – until the whole decidua is homogeneously reflective, so that the three lines can no longer be delineated (Figure 13). When this pattern was present at 6–9 days after the surge of luteinizing hormone (LH), the endometrium was found to be normal in 82% according to histological criteria, whereas this was the case in less than 50% with the examination of hypoechogenic ultrasound patterns[19].

Under hormonal treatment also, there was a good correlation between development of a hyperechogenic endometrium and histological changes of the stroma in the second half of the cycle[20]. Development of the echogenicity is attributed to the increase of mucus and glycogen and to the increase of ultrasound interfaces caused by the gyrated glands[16] as well as do the edematous stroma reaction[20]. During the secretory phase, there is no significant change of endometrial thickness[15,17]. Some authors have noticed a maximum of 14 mm in the mid-secretory phase[16]. The endometrial volume in a normal spontaneous cycle, calculated from the three diameters perpendicular to one another, is 1.6 ± 0.4 ml during the proliferative stage, and 3.6 ± 0.8 ml during the secretory stage[16].

Shortly before menstruation, decrease of the mucosa diameter occurs. During menstruation, the uterine cavity can be filled with blood and shed decidua tissue. It presents a complex struc-

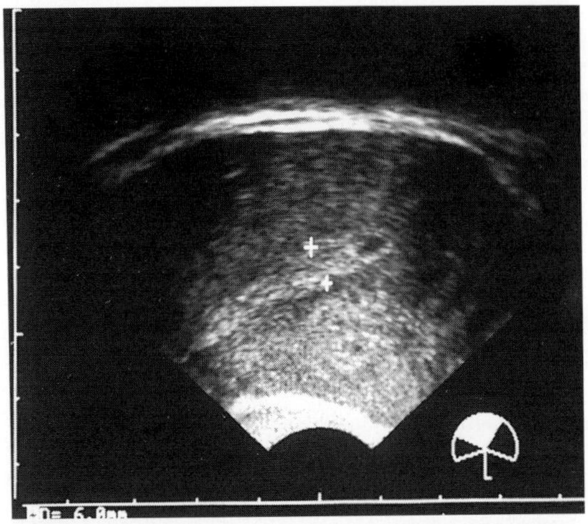

Figure 14 Endometrium at the time of menstruation (diameter, D = 6 mm)

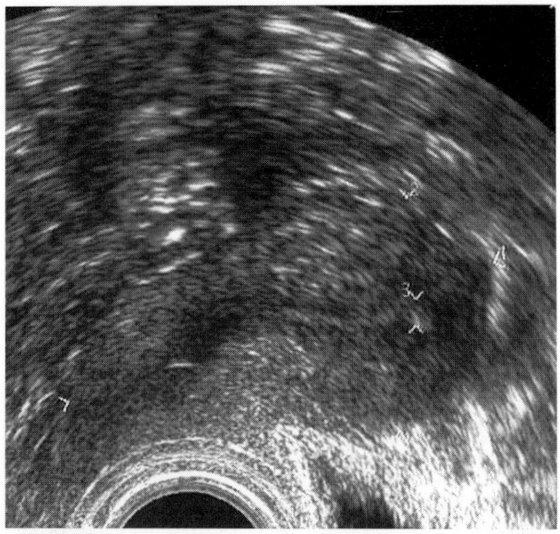

Figure 15 Atrophic uterus with narrow endometrium in the postmenopause (diameters, D3 = 4 mm, D2 = 31 mm, D1 = 63 mm)

ture with echoless and hyper-reflective components (Figure 14).

The endometrium in postmenopausal women

After the menopause, decrease of ovarian estrogen production leads to atrophy of the endometrium. In consequence the endometrial band is sonographically narrow and the echogenic line of the uterine cavity often cannot be visualized (Figure 15). The endometrium could not be localized in 7% of postmenopausal women without a bleeding disorder[12] or 10% of women with histologically detected atrophic endometrium[21]. In addition, shadowing arising from myomas or arteriosclerosis can make visualization more difficult. Echotexture of the endometrium is usually more echogenic than the surrounding myometrium. In a study with 279 assessable endometria, 85% were more echogenic and 9% less echogenic than the myometrium and 6% showed both reflection patterns[12].

The poorly echogenic myometrial zone round the endometrium is frequently absent in the postmenopause. The endometrial thickness in the postmenopause is 2–4 mm, with a considerable scatter range of 0–10 mm, and consequently there are different limiting values for the normal state in the literature (Table 6). Endometrial thickness correlates with body weight[12]. Postmenopausal

Table 6 Vaginosonographic standard values for thickness of the endometrium in asymptomatic postmenopausal women, and limiting values (mm), above which the endometrium was classified as suspicious

Author	*n*	*Value*	*Range*	*Normal limiting value*	*Proportion above limiting value in normal histology* (%)
Fleischer *et al.* (1990)[16]	–	–	4–8	< 10	–
Schoenfeld *et al.* (1990)[23]	–	–	5–8	8	–
Osmers *et al.* (1990)[22]	205	–	–	< 8*	0.5
Lin *et al.* (1991)[26]	57†	4‡	0–15	10	11
Varner *et al.* (1991)[24]	63**	3.2††	< 2–8	< 5	16
Andolf *et al.* (1993)[12]	300	2.3 ± 1.8‡‡	0–10	< 5	7

*Values given by the author converted into thickness including both layers; †transvaginal and/or transabdominal sonography; ‡median; **included women with hormonal substitution therapy; ††mean; ‡‡mean ± SD from 279 measurable endometria

women, who have bleeding after taking progesterone, on average have a thicker endometrium than do women with a negative gestagen test[25]. The intensity and interval of the withdrawal bleeding also correlate with the endometrial thickness. Women with pure estrogen replacement therapy more frequently have endometrial thicknesses exceeding normal values[26].

In about 10% of cases, there are fluid pools in the uterine cavity, which are independent of endometrial thickness and normally do not surpass volumes of 1 ml, with no further increase[26]. These are possibly secretion pools not able to drain out, as a result of cervical stenosis.

References

1. Mendelson, E. B., Bohm-Velez, M., Joseph, N. and Neimann, H. L. (1988). Gynecologic imaging; comparison of transabdominal and transvaginal sonography. *Radiology*, **166**, 321–4
2. Tessler, F. N., Schiller, V. L., Perrella, R. R., Sutherland, M. L. and Grant, E. G. (1989). Transabdominal versus endovaginal pelvic sonography. Prospective study. *Radiology*, **170**, 553–6
3. Mitchell, D. G., Schonholz, L., Hilpert, P. L., Pennell, R. G., Blum, L. and Rifkin, M. D. (1990). Zones of the uterus: discrepancy between US an MR images. *Radiology*, **174**, 827–31
4. Hata, K., Nishigaki, A., Makihara, K., Takamiya, O., Hata, T. and Kitao, M. (1989). Ultrasonic evaluation of the normal uterus in the neonata. *J. Perinat. Med.*, **17**, 313–17
5. Pelzer, V. (1991). Der Stellenwert der Ultrasonographie in der Kinder- und Jugendgynäkologie. *Gynäkologe*, **24**, 91–6
6. Orsini, L. F., Salardi, S., Pilu, G., Bovicelli, L. and Cacciari, E. (1984). Pelvic organs in premenarcheal girls: real-time ultrasonography. *Radiology*, **153**, 113–16
7. Hein, P. R., Eskes, T. K. A. B., Stolte, L. A. M., Braaksma, J. F., Janssens, J. and Hoek, J. M. (1973). The influence of steroids on uterine motility in the non-pregnant human uterus. In Josimovich, J. B. (ed.) *Uterine Contraction – Side-effects of Steroidal Contraceptives*, pp. 107–40. (New York: Wiley and Sons)
8. de Vries, K., Lyons, K. E. A., Ballard, G., Levi, C. S. and Lindsay, D. J. (1990). Contractions of the inner third of the myometrium. *Am. J. Obstet. Gynecol.*, **162**, 679–82
9. Becker, R., Entezami, M., Hese, S., Vollert, W., Loy, V. and Weitzel, H. K. (1994). Gynäkologische Sonographie II. Normalwerte der standardisierten Uterusbiometrie. *Ultraschall Klin. Prax.*, **8**, 241–7
10. Saxton, D. W., Farquhar, C. M., Rae, T., Beard, R.W., Anderson, M.C. and Wadsworth, J. (1990). Accuracy of ultrasound measurements of female pelvic organs. *Br. J. Obstet. Gynaecol*, **97**, 695–9
11. Plätt, J. F., Bree, R. L. and Davidson, D. (1990). Ultrasound of the normal nongravid uterus: correlation with gross and histopathology. *J. Clin. Ultrasound*, **18**, 15–19
12. Andolf, E., Dahlander, K. and Aspenberg, P. (1993). Ultrasonic thickness of the endometrium correlated to body weight in asymptomatic postmenopausal women. *Obstet. Gynecol.*, **82**, 936–40
13. Fleischer, A. C., Kalemeris, G. C., Machin, J. E., Entman, S. S. and James, E. (1986). Sonographic depiction of normal and abnormal endometrium with histopathologic correlation. *J. Ultrasound Med.*, **5**, 445–52
14. Forrest, T. S., Elyaderani, M. K., Muilenburg, M. I., Bewtra, C., Kable, W. T. and Sullivan, P. (1988), Cyclic endometrial changes: US assessment with histologic correlation. *Radiology*, **167**, 233–7
15. Randall, J. M., Fisk, N. M., McTavish, A. and Templeton, A. A. (1989). Transvaginal ultrasonic assessment of endometrial growth in spontaneous and hyperstimulated menstrual cycles. *Br. J. Obstet. Gynaecol.*, **96**, 954–9
16. Fleischer, A. C., Gordon, A. N. and Entman, S. S. (1990). Transvaginal scanning of the endometrium. *J. Clin. Ultrasound*, **18**, 337–49
17. Bakos, O., Lundkvist, Ö. and Bergh, T. (1993). Transvaginal sonographic evaluation of endometrial growth and texture in spontaneous ovulatory cycles – a descriptive study. *Hum. Reprod.*, **8**, 799–806
18. Ueno, J., Oehninger, S., Bryski, R. G., Acosta, A. A., Philput, C. B. and Muasher, S. J. (1991). Ultrasonic appearance of the endometrium in natural and stimulated *in-vitro* fertilization cycles and its correlation with outcome. *Hum Reprod.*, **6**, 901–4
19. Doherty, C. M., Silver, B., Binor, Z., Wood Molo, M. and Radwanska, E. (1993). Transvaginal ultrasonography and the assessment of luteal phase endometrium. *Am. J. Obstet. Gynecol.*, **168**, 1702–9
20. Grunfeld, L., Walker, B., Bergh, P. A., Sandler, B.,

Hofmann, G. and Navor, D. (1991). High-resolution endovaginal ultrasonography of the endometrium: a noninvasive test for endometrial adequacy. *Obstet. Gynecol.*, **78**, 200–4
21. Granberg, S., Wikland, M., Karlsson, B., Nordström, A. and Friberg, L. G. (1991). Endometrial thickness as measured by endovaginal ultrasound for identifying endometrial abnormality. *Am. J. Obstet. Gynecol.*, **164**, 47–52
22. Osmers, R., Völksen, M. and Schauer, A. (1990). Vaginosonography for early detection of endometrial carcinoma? *Lancet*, **335**, 1569–71
23. Schoenfeld, A., Levavi, H., Hirsch, M., Pardo, J. and Ovadia, J. (1990). Transvaginal sonography in postmenopausal women. *J. Clin. Ultrasound*, **18**, 350–8
24. Varner, R. E., Sparks, J. M., Cameron, C. D., Roberts, L. L. and Soong, S.-J. (1991). Transvaginal sonography of the endometrium in postmenopausal women. *Obstet. Gynecol.*, **78**, 195–9
25. Pansini, F., De Paoli, D., Serra, M. M., Campobasso, C., Levato, F. and Fuilini, D. (1992). Combined use of progesterone challenge test and endometrium thickness evaluated by transvaginal ultrasonography in the preventive management of postmenopausal women. *Gynecol. Obstet. Invest.*, **34**, 237–9
26. Lin, M. C., Gosin, B. B., Wolf, S. I., Feldesman, M. R., Stuenkel, C. A., Braly, P. S. and Pretorius, D. H. (1991). Endometrial thickness after menopause: effect of hormone replacement. *Radiology*, **180**, 427–32

Sonographic evaluation of the cervix uteri

2

A. Suren, J. Puchta and R. Osmers

The cervix uteri with the cervical canal constitutes the lower third of the uterus. The relationship between the length of the corpus uteri and the cervix varies during the lifetime of a woman. Uterine growth develops, with a corpus/cervix ratio of 1:3 in childhood, reaching its final maturity with a ratio of 3:1. In the infantile uterus, the cervix accounts for two-thirds of the uterine length. On the other hand, a hypoplastic uterus is proportioned like a normal uterus, but with a total size below normal.

The cervix is shaped like a cylinder and consists of fibrous and elastic connective tissue and smooth muscle fibers. The cervical canal leads with its proximal end, the os internum, into the uterine cavity and with its distal end, the os externum, into the upper part of the vagina. The cervical canal is covered by a monostratified blennogenic epithelium, which is reactive to ovarian hormones.

The cervix uteri and cervical secretions are important for the following regenerative functions. First, the cervix serves as a depot for spermatozoa. It protects against the acid vaginal secretion and supplies energy for the spermatozoa. In addition, it serves as a reservoir, subsequently allowing the migration of spermatozoa into the uterine cavity.

These mechanisms are under hormonal influence. Estrogens induce the production of mucus, which is essential for sperm ascension. Storage of the spermatozoa in the cervical canal is improved by increasing the number and the size of the crypts[1]. A decrease in mucus production, due to cervicitis or to conization, with subsequent shortening of the cervical canal, can be the cause of cervical sterility.

When the cervix is viewed, attention should be paid to inclusion of the os internum and os externum as part of the image. The fibrous part of

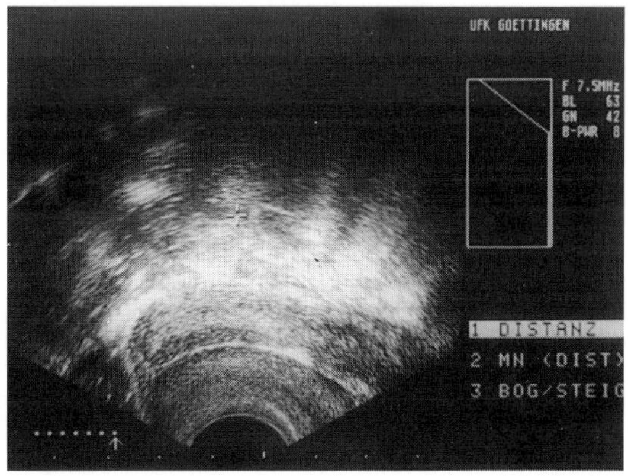

Figure 1 Normal cervix (longitudinal section). The echogenic cervical canal is well outlined

the cervix uteri shows a medium-level echotexture. Delimitation of the cervix from the surroundings can be recognized by hyperreflective lines (Figure 1). In the horizontal section, the cervix appears oval. As with the endometrium, the cervix shows changes that depend on the menstrual cycle. During menstruation, the echogenic stripe of bleeding can be viewed. The sonographic picture of the cervix postmenstrually does not change until the beginning of the mid-follicular phase. The anterior and posterior wall of the cervical canal are adjacent to one another and appear as an echogenic line. Under the increasing estrogen effect in the late follicular phase – around the time of ovulation – a hypoechogenic or echoless stripe can be observed between the os internum and os externum. In the physiological cycle, this stripe reaches its maximum breadth of 4–5 mm by the time of ovulation (Figure 2). Thus, mid-cyclic cervical mucus can be viewed sonographically[2].

After rupture of the follicle, the hypoechogenic stripe has soon receded by the time of the second

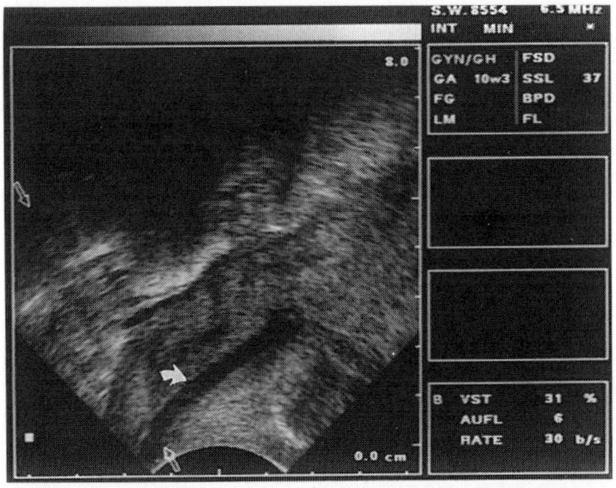

Figure 2 Longitudinal section showing mid-cyclic opening of the cervical canal (white arrow)

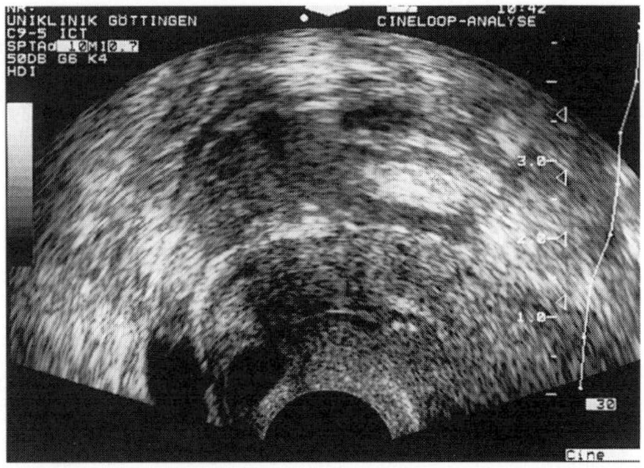

Figure 3 Cervix with ovulum Nabothi in the anterior labium of the os uteri with dorsal echo enhancement

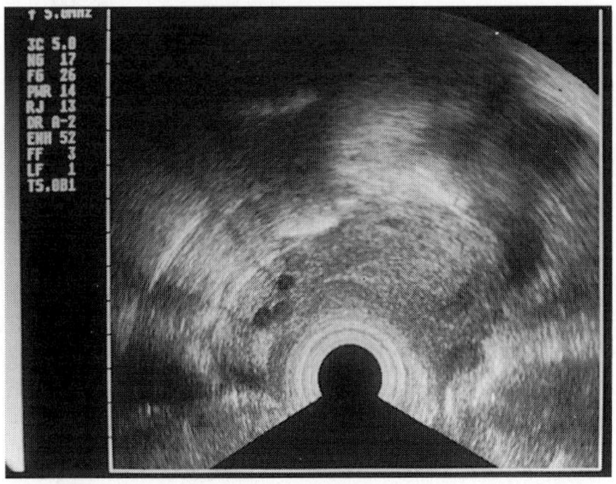

Figure 4 Longitudinal section of uterus with cervical cysts

postovulatory day, i.e. the cervical canal is closed again. This sequence of events is observed both in spontaneous cycles and in cycles under hormonal replacement therapy[3]. Hill and colleagues[2] were able to detect cervical mucus with transabdominal ultrasound in only 5% of cycles treated with human menopausal gonadotropin (hMG) or clomiphene. The sonographically measured volumes of the mucus were independent of the serum estradiol levels[4]. Eppel and associates[3] were able to delimit the cervical canal clearly – with transvaginal ultrasound – in about four-fifths of all patients who had received clomiphene/hMG therapy before *in vitro* fertilization treatment. In some cases there was no preovulatory transformation of the ectocervix, i.e. there was no cervical plug, although serum estradiol levels were high enough. Thus, mucus production in the endo- and ectocervix can differ visibly.

SONOGRAPHIC FEATURES OF BENIGN LESIONS

Small, oval hypoechogenic areas in the cervical wall, with a dorsal echo enhancement, correspond with the histological findings of retention cysts (Figures 3 and 4). Cervical polyps appear as plump, hypoechogenic structures in the dilated cervical canal.

Cervical myomas are rare and account for only 8% of all uterine myomas (Figure 5). The cervix appears distended, and the normal echotexture has disappeared. The capsule of the myoma can be recognized from the presence of a hyperechogenic line. According to the proportion of degenerative changes, myomas vary considerably in their appearance. Whereas calcified myomas present themselves as hyperechogenic, necrotizing myomas present as hypoechogenic and echoless areas. Myomas with rapid growth and good vascularization, however, present themselves as homogeneously hypoechogenic.

In a double uterus there are two cervical canals.

Occasionally (0.5% of all ectopic pregnancies) implantation of the blastocyst occurs intracervically. With transvaginal sonography, the trophoblast appears as an echogenic ring structure in the area of the cervix.

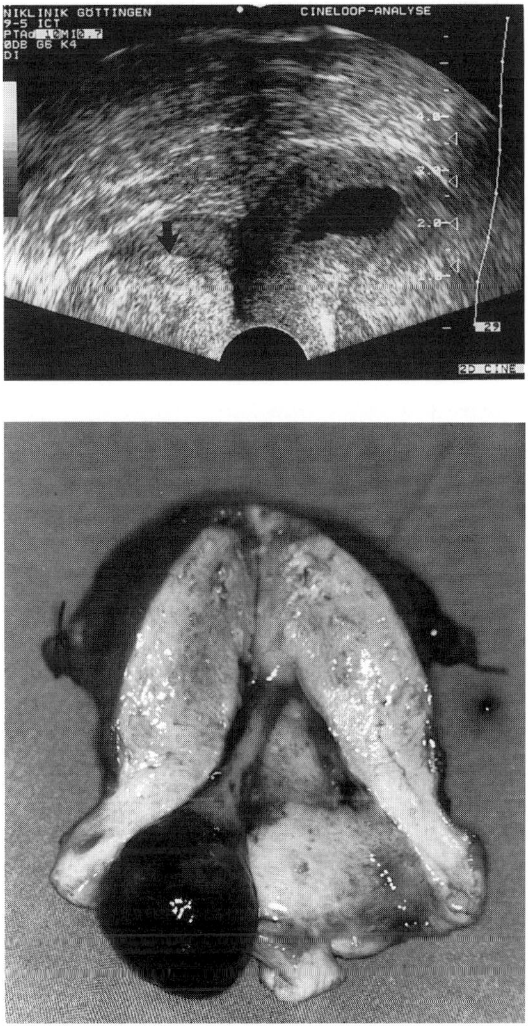

Figure 5 Longitudinal section of uterus (above) with hematometra and cervical myoma in statu nascendi (black arrow), and specimen (below) of the cervical myoma

After Cesarean section, the scar tissue of the uterotomy is seen as an irregularly outlined, hyperechogenic area in the region of the posterior wall of the isthmus uteri. Wound dehiscences can also be viewed; they appear as triangular echoless areas (Figure 6).

SONOGRAPHIC FEATURES OF MALIGNANT LESIONS

Cervical cancer is the most common cancer of the female genital tract, accounting for approximately 35–50% of all genital malignancies. In some countries, however, the incidence of cervical carcinoma exceeds – to an increasing degree – the incidence of endometrial cancer. Of all persons affected, 7% are younger than 30; it is most frequent between the age of 45 and 55. The fact that today about one-third of all cervical cancers are detected at stage I and approximately one-third at stage II is due to screening measures using Papanicolaou smears of the cervix. With the help of early check-ups, 80–90% of paraneoplastic changes can be detected. Nevertheless, the proportion of 11–13% of false-negative results demands supplementary screening methods[5].

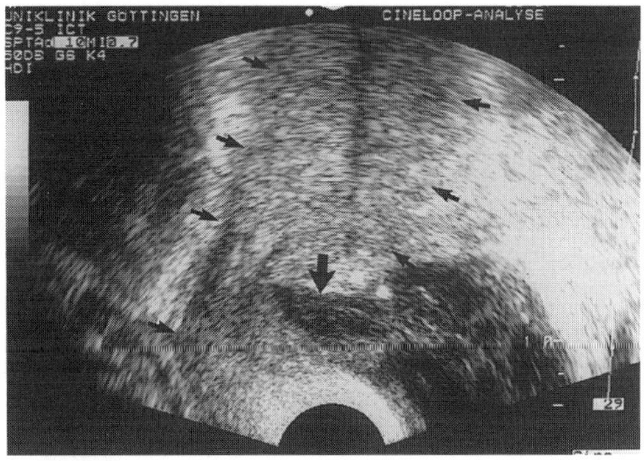

Figure 6 Wound dehiscence (large black arrow) with hematoma after Cesarean section. Uterus indicated by small black arrows

The prognosis of manifest cervical cancer depends on the tumor volume at the time of diagnosis. The decision on which treatment to choose depends on the FIGO stage, which is based on inspection, palpation and surgical staging. Each of these methods has its limits, however. A tumor growing endocervically will not be detected by inspection; a tumor at stage Ia/Ib cannot be palpated, and with a tumor at stage Ib/IIb, being treated by conization, there is a risk that the tumor will be cut into, particularly when there is ignorance of the exact localization and tumor size. Currently, development of vaginal and rectal high-resolution probes enables us to classify, more exactly, in the course of pretherapeutic staging examinations, the localization of the tumor, its size and possible extension onto the pelvic side wall, parametria or adjacent organs. Even preinvasive changes of the epithe-

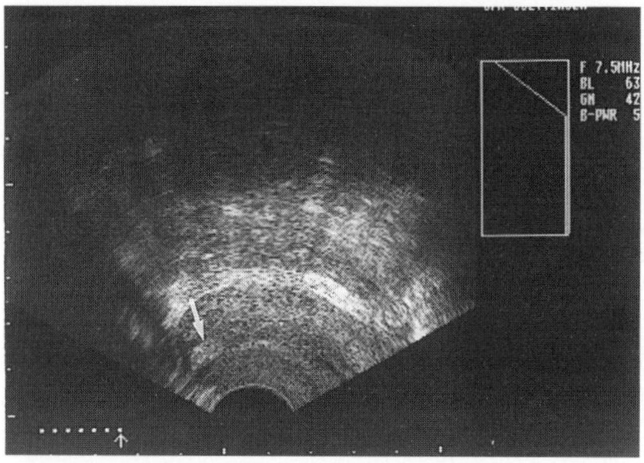

Figure 7 Longitudinal section showing cervix with echogenic mass (arrow) corresponding with a carcinoma *in situ*

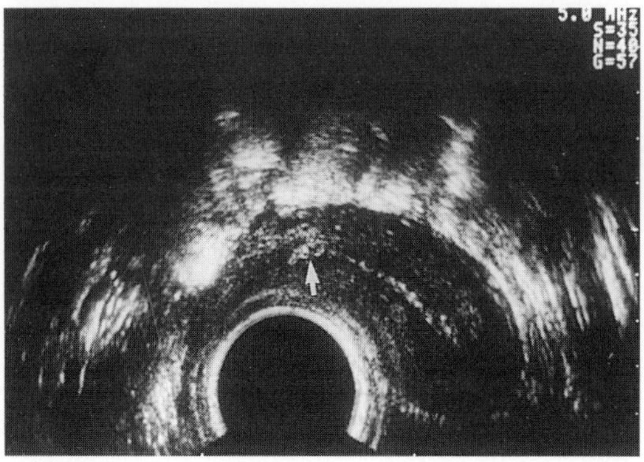

Figure 8 Longitudinal section showing cervix with echogenic mass (arrow) corresponding with a carcinoma *in situ*

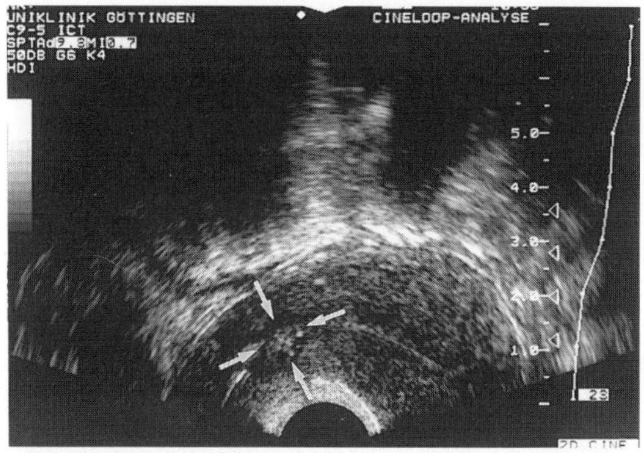

Figure 9 Longitudinal section of the uterus, showing cervical carcinoma Ia (arrows)

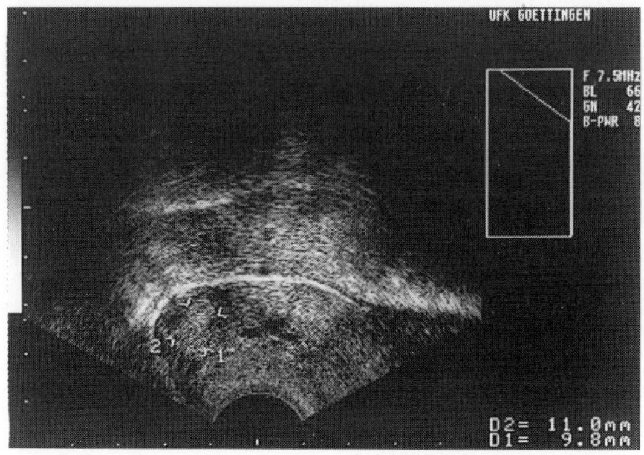

Figure 10 Longitudinal section of the cervix, showing cervical carcinoma Ib (arrowheads)

lium like PAP IIID/IV, that will be treated by conization and dilatation and curettage, and which show the histological features of a carcinoma *in situ*, present a suspicious echo-texture in the cervix[6] (Figures 7 and 8). Because of its low sensitivity and specifity, sonography alone is no screening method of early endometrial carcinoma, but it can – in conjunction with cytology – contribute to an improvement of downsize and therapy. Localization of areas in the cytologically suspicious cervix can be helpful when deciding on the depth of incision of a conization sample.

Besides producing morphological changes such as ballooning, cervical cancer leads to an alteration of the normal reflection patterns of the cervix. In addition to heterogeneously contoured hypo- or hyperechogenic areas, non-homogeneous lesions can often be viewed (Figures 9–11). If the epithelium is involved, the bright reflection lines of the cervical canal are fuzzy or interrupted or they cannot be viewed at all. If the tumor extends to the environment, the mainly hypoechogenic tumor masses can be viewed as irregularly protruding, solid pegs. Larger abscess cavities, which are a result of tumor necrosis, frequently show an increased echogenicity, provided there are aerogenic micro-organisms forming small bubbles of gas. Infiltration into the urinary bladder can be visualized by both transvaginal and transabdominal sonography, if the

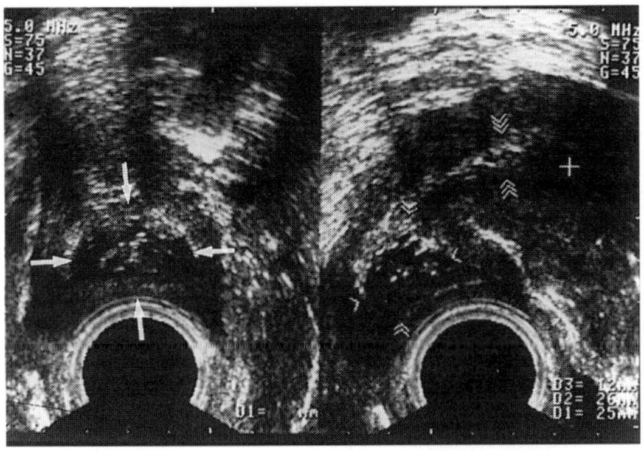

Figure 11 Uterine transverse section (left) and longitudinal section (right) showing tumor crater (arrows)

bladder is filled. If there are immobile intestinal loops that cannot be moved along the posterior wall of the uterus, invasion of the bowel should be suspected. This requires preoperative bowel diagnostics.

Preoperative detection of involvement of the parametria often turns out to be difficult, as exact differentiation between cancerous and inflammatory infiltration is not possible[7-11]. It has not been possible up to the present time to attain this differentiation by means of rectosonography[12-14]. The situation is similar for the detection of pelvic and paraortic lymph nodes; these cannot be visualized sonographically, due to bowel gas superposition. In these cases, computerized tomography appears to be more exact than ultrasound examination[15,16]. The use of sonography is more successful in detecting tumorous urinary obstruction or hydronephrosis and in excluding tumor recurrence with follow-up treatment.

References

1. Insler, V., Glezerman, M. and Gaton, E. (1985). Der zervikale Faktor als Sterilitätsursache: Pathophysiologie und klinische Aspekte. In Distler, W. and Hofmann, N. (eds.) *Fertilitätsstörungen*, pp. 53–61. (Stuttgart: Thieme)
2. Hill, L.M., Coulam, C.B., Kislak, S.L., Peterson, G.S. and Runco, C.J. (1987). Sonographic evaluation of the cervix during ovulation induction. *Am. J. Obstet. Gynecol.*, **157**, 1170–4
3. Eppel, W., Schurz, B., Knogler, W., Huber, J. and Reinhold, E. (1987). Sonographische Darstellung funktioneller Zervixveränderungen im Rahmen der Sterilitätsabklärung. In Hansmann, M., Koischwitz, D., Lutz, H. and Trier, H. G. (eds.) *Ultraschalldiagnostik 86*, pp. 306–8. (Berlin, Heidelberg, New York: Springer)
4. Deichert, U. and Michaels, W. (1993) Zyklische Veränderungen am Uterus. In Deichert, U., Duda, V. and Schlief, R. (eds.) *Funktionelle Sonographie in Gynäkologie und Reproduktionsmedizin*, pp. 43–69. (Berlin: Springer)
5. Hilgarth, M. (1986). Qualitätssicherung der gynäkologischen Eytologie. In Hilgarth, M. and Szalay, L. (eds.) *Farbatlas der gynäkologischen Zytodiagnostik*, p. 80. (München: Hans Marseille Verlag)
6. Suren, A., Dietrich, M., Osmers, M. and Osmers, R. (1994). Transvaginosonography in patients with pathological cervical exfoliative cytology or histologically verified cervical carcinoma. *Int. J. Gynecol. Obstet.*, **47**, in press
7. Bernadino, M. E. and Dodd, G. D. (1981). Imaging of the pelvic contents in the female oncologic patient. *Cancer*, **48**, 504
8. Fleischer, A. C., Walsh, J. W., Jones, H. W., Shaff, A. E. and James, A. E. (1982). Sonographic evaluation of pelvic masses. *Radiol. Clin. N. Am.*, **20**, 397
9. Hansmann, M. (1985). Pathologie des Genitales. In Hansmann, M. B., Hackelöer, B. J. and Staudach, A. (eds.) *Ultraschalldiagnostik in Geburtshilfe und Gynäkologie. Lehrbuch und Atlas*, pp. 367–84. (Berlin: Springer)
10. Kurtz, A. B., Rubin, C. S., Kramer, F. L. and Goldberg, B. B. (1979). Ultrasound evaluation of the posterior pelvic compartment. *Radiology*, **132**, 677
11. Sanders, R. C. (1984). Ultrasound in pelvic malignancy. In Steel, W. B. and Cochrane, W. J. (eds.) *Gynecologic Ultrasound*. (New York: Churchill Livingstone)
12. Bernaschek, G. and Janisch, H. (1983). Eine Methode zur Objektivierung des Parametrienbefundes beim Zervixkarzinom. *Geburtshilf. Frauenheilk.*, **43**, 498
13. Blake, D. (1979). Transrectal ultrasonography in the evaluation of cervical carcinoma. *Obstet. Gynecol.*, **53**, 105

14. Zaritzky, D., Blake, D., Willard, J. and Resnick, M. (1979). Transrectal ultrasonography in the evaluation of cervical carcinoma. *Obstet. Gynecol.*, **53**, 105
15. Ginaldi, S., Wallace, S., Jing, B. S. and Bernardino, M. E. (1981). Carcinoma of the cervix: lymphangiography and computed tomography. *Am. J. Roentgenol.*, **136**, 1087
16. Walsh, J. W., Amendola, M. A., Konerding, K. F., Tisnado, J. and Hazra, T. A. (1980) Computed tomographic detection of pelvic and inguinal lymph node metastases from primary and recurrent pelvic malignant disease. *Radiology*, **137**, 157

Sonographic evaluation of the cervix uteri in pregnancy

3

M. Dietrich and R. Osmers

NORMAL SONOGRAPHIC FINDINGS

Assessment of the cervical status is an important component of obstetric monitoring, aiding in the detection and management of cervical incompetence and preterm labor.

The average size of the uterine cervix of a non-pregnant woman is about 2.5 cm in length, and up to 6 cm in length during pregnancy[1]. However, characteristic changes can be observed during the course of pregnancy. Kushnir and Podobnik and their colleagues demonstrated that cervical length increases progressively up to 20–25 weeks' gestation and then decreases significantly at 31–37 weeks' gestation[2,3]. Beginning at 32 weeks, a significant cervical shortening can be observed[2,4]. According to these authors, the mean cervical length for each gestational age is not significantly different between primigravid/primiparous women on the one hand and multigravid/multiparous women on the other hand[2,4]. Pfersmann and associates[5], however, demonstrated that, from 35 weeks onward, cervical shortening is more pronounced in multiparous women. In the 30th gestational week, an average cervical length of 4.0 cm can be observed, whereas in the 40th week of gestation, the average length is 2.5 cm[5].

Digital examination is the most common method of assessing the cervix in pregnancy and has long been the 'gold' standard. Its accuracy, however, has been questioned. Examiners tend to underestimate cervical length, as they are not able to palpate the supravaginal portion of the cervix, which represents up to one-half of the cervix[6–9]. Böhmer and co-workers[10] found an increasing variability of digital examination with increasing cervical incompetence.

In contrast, transvaginal ultrasonography has been demonstrated to be a valid and reproducible method of cervical assessment in pregnancy[7]. It allows measurement of the entire length of the cervix[7], visualization of the internal os[11] and detection of placenta previa[12]. Cervical length is measured along the endocervical canal from the internal to the external os. The base of the internal os is identified as the apex of the V-shaped membrane covering the cervix[9] (Figure 1).

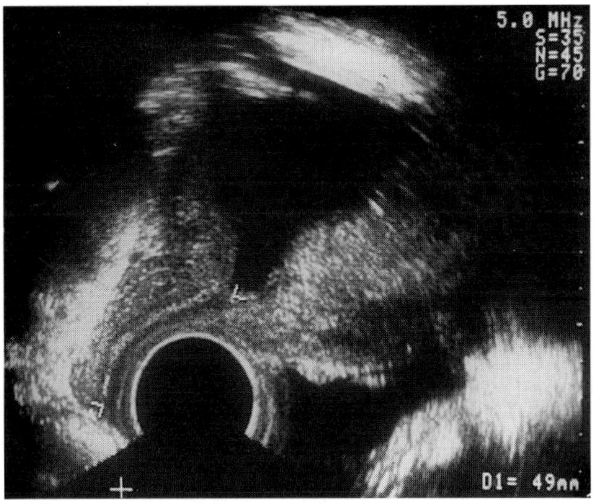

Figure 1 Ultrasound scan in primigravida in the 25th gestational week. Cervical length is measured along the endocervical canal from the internal os to the external os

SONOGRAPHIC FEATURES OF CERVICAL INCOMPETENCE

Cervical incompetence is characterized by dilatation and shortening of the cervix prior to the 37th gestational week with or without premature labor[3,10,13]. Bengtsson defined cervical incompetence as primary failure of the uterine cervix to retain an intrauterine pregnancy, resulting in preterm dilatation of the cervix in the absence of uterine contractions, often accompanied by premature rupture of membranes[14]. Early detection of cervical incompetence is of considerable importance for the prevention of miscarriage or premature delivery.

In addition to the measurement of total cervical length by transvaginal sonographic assessment, changes at the level of the internal os, such as endocervical dilatation and membrane protrusion, can be viewed[9,15,16]. According to Bartolucci and colleagues[15], dilatation of the endocervical canal must be considered if the maximum caliber exceeds 1 cm.

Michaels and associates[9] divided membrane protrusion into two degrees. Cervical nippling was described as membrane protrusion through the internal os for an arbitrarily defined distance of <6 mm. Membrane herniation represented protrusion of the membranes through the internal os for a distance of >6 mm.

An advanced variant of membrane protrusion is represented by the so-called 'hourglass membranes', a frank prolapse of the amniotic sac through the moderately dilated internal os[17] (Figures 2–4).

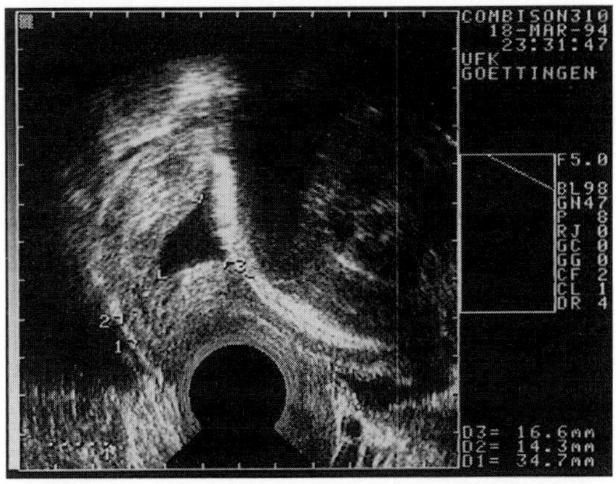

Figure 2 Ultrasound scan in primigravida in the 32nd gestational week, showing endocervical dilatation and membrane protrusion into the cervical canal

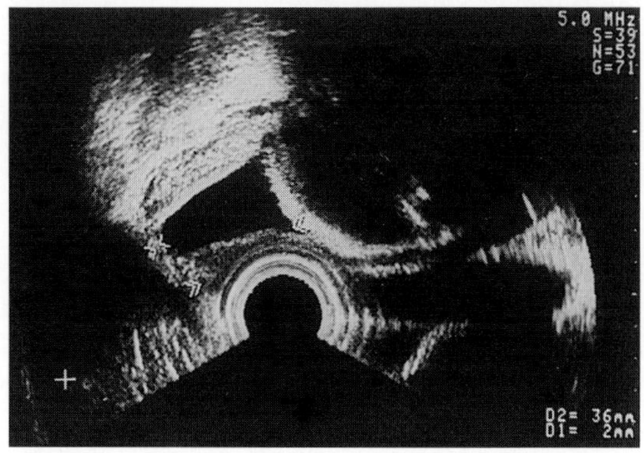

Figure 3 Ultrasound scan in multigravid/multiparous woman in the 34th gestational week, showing bulging of the membranes into the cervical canal with dilatation of the external os

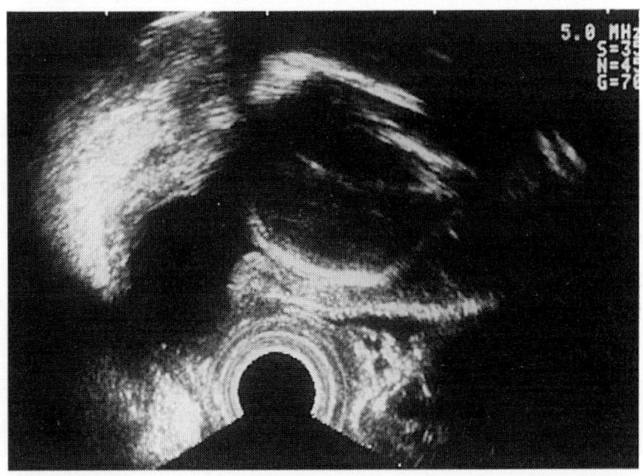

Figure 4 Ultrasound scan in primigravida in the 33rd gestational week, showing 'hourglass membrane': prolapse of the membranes through the moderately dilated internal os

SONOGRAPHIC EVALUATION AFTER CERCLAGE

The question of whether a patient should undergo cervical cerclage as prophylaxis against premature delivery due to cervical incompetence is controversial[9,16,18].

Höckel and colleages demonstrated that only patients with premature cervical ripening before the 25th week of gestation and patients with an 'open cervix' *and* a history of miscarriage, abortion or premature delivery will benefit from cerclage placement[19]. Serial sonographic evaluation of the cervix during pregnancy allows detection of a progressive decrease in cervical length and dilatation of the internal os and therefore may provide objective grounds for or against the need for cerclage[6].

When operative treatment has been performed, the value of transvaginal sonography lies in a follow-up examination, demonstrating the localization of the band used for cerclage and the configuration of the internal os (Figures 5 and 6).

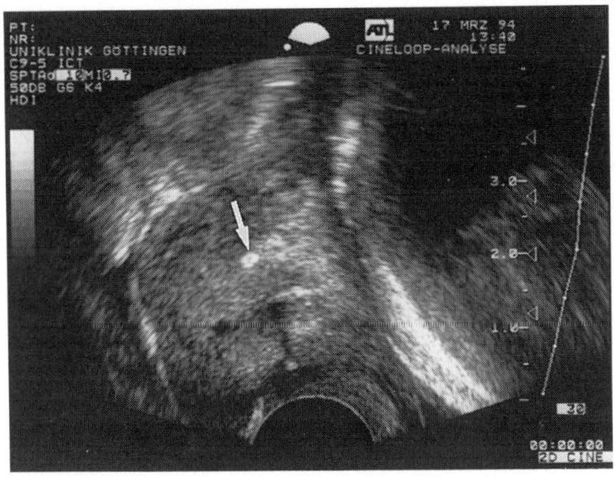

Figure 5 Ultrasound scan in multigravid/multiparous woman in the 29th gestational week, showing localization of the band of cerclage (arrow)

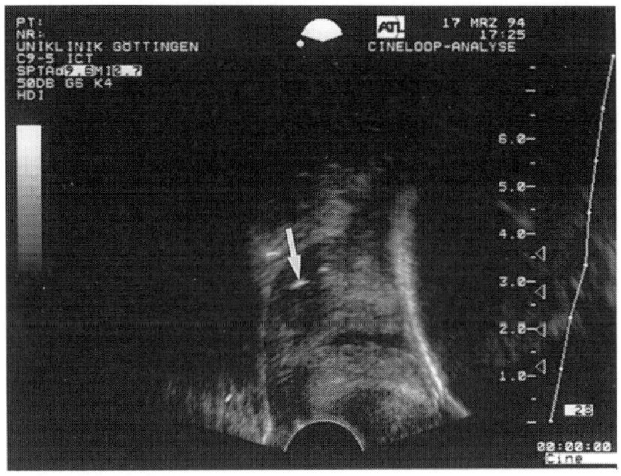

Figure 6 Ultrasound scan in primigravid woman in the 34th gestational week, showing non-optimal localization of the band of cerclage (arrow)

References

1. Zemlyn, S. (1981). The length of the uterine cervix and its significance. *J. Clin. Ultrasound*, **9**, 267–9
2. Kushnir, O., Vigil, D. A., Izquierdo, L., Schift, M. and Curet L. B. (1990). Vaginal ultrasonographic assessment of cervical length changes during normal pregnancy. *Am. J. Obstet. Gynecol.*, **162**, 991–3
3. Podobnik, M., Bulic, M., Smiljanic, N. and Bistricki, J. (1988). Ultrasonography in the detection of cervical incompetency. *J. Clin. Ultrasound*, **13**, 383–91
4. Ayers, J. W. T., De Grood, R. M., Compton, A. A., Barclay, M. and Ansbacher, R. (1988). Sonographic evaluation of cervical length in pregnancy: diagnosis and management of preterm cervical effacement in patients at risk for premature delivery. *Obstet. Gynecol.*, **71**, 939–44
5. Pfersmann, C., Deutinger, J. and Bernaschek, G. (1986). Die Zervixlänge gegen Ende der Schwangerschaft – eine sonographische Studie. *Geburtshilf. Frauenheilk.*, **46**, 213–14
6. Chung, T. K. H., Haines, C. J., Kong, D., Woo, W. K. and Rogers, M. S. (1993). Transvaginal sonography in the diagnosis and management of cervical incompetence. *Gynecol. Obstet. Invest.*, **36**, 59–61
7. Jackson, G. M., Ludmir, J. and Bader, T. J. (1992). The accuracy of digital examination and ultrasound in the evaluation of cervical length. *Obstet. Gynecol.*, **79**, 214–18
8. Lim, B. H., Mahmood, T. A., Smith, N. C. and Beat, I. (1992). A prospective comparative study of transvaginal ultrasonography digital examination for cervical assessment in the third trimester of pregnancy. *Clin. Ultrasound*, **20**, 599–603
9. Michaels, W. H., Montgomery, C., Karo, J., Temple, J., Ager, J. and Olson, J. (1986). Ultrasound differentiation of the competent from the incompetent cervix: prevention of preterm delivery. *Am. J. Obstet. Gynecol.*, **154**, 537–46
10. Böhmer, S., Degenhardt, F., Gerlach, C., Behrens, O. and Mühlhaus, K. (1989). Vaginalsonographie als Untersuchungsverfahren zur Beurteilung der Cervixinsuffizienz. *Ultraschall*, **10**, 19–24
11. Brown, J. E., Thieme, G. A., Shah, D. M., Fleischer, A. C. and Boehm, F. H. (1986). Transabdominal and transvaginal endosonography: evaluation of the cervix and lower uterine segment in pregnancy. *Arch. J. Obstet. Gynecol.*, **155**, 721–6
12. Farine, D., Fox, H. E., Jakobsen, S. and Timor-Tritsch, H. E. (1988). Vaginal ultrasound for diagnosis of placenta previa. *Am. J. Obstet. Gynecol.*, **159**, 566–9
13. Böhmer, S., Degenhardt, F., Gerlach, C., Jagla, K. and Schnieder, J. (1989). Vaginalsonographie versus vaginaler Tastbefund: erste Erfahrungen bei 120 schwangeren Frauen mit Verdacht auf Zervixinsuffizienz. *Z. Geburtsh. Perinat.*, **193**, 115–23
14. Bengtsson, L. P. (1968). Cervical insufficiency. *Acta Obstet. Gynecol. Scand.*, **47** (Suppl. 1)
15. Bartolucci, L., Hill, W. C., Katz, M., Gill, P. J. and Kitzmiller, J. L. (1984). Ultrasonography in preterm labor. *Am. J. Obstet. Gynecol.*, **149**, 52–6
16. Michaels, W. H., Schreiber, F. R., Padgett, R. J.,

Ager, J. and Pieper, D. (1991). Ultrasound surveillance of the cervix in twin gestations: management of cervical incompetency. *Obstet. Gynecol.*, **78**, 739–44
17. Harris, R. D. and Barth, R. A. (1993). Sonography of the gravid uterus and placenta: current concepts. *Am. J. Radiol.*, **160**, 455–65
18. Jofte, G. M., Del Valle, G. O., Izquierdo, L. A., Gilson, G. J., Smith, J. F., Chatterjee, M. S. and Curet, L. B. (1992). Diagnosis of cervical change in pregnancy by means of transvaginal ultrasonography. *Am. J. Obstet. Gynecol.*, **166**, 896–900
19. Höckel, M., Krämer, S. and Lippold, R. (1987). Vorzeitige Zervixreifung – operative oder konservative Therapie? *Z. Geburtsh. Perinat.*, **191**, 105–14

Sonographic depiction of the uterus 4

A. Suren, J. Puchta and R. Osmers

MORPHOLOGICAL FINDINGS IN THE PREMENOPAUSAL ENDOMETRIUM

The endometrium consists of a pars functionalis (with a superficial pars compacta and a pars spongiosa lying below), the regulation and function of which is subject to ovarian hormones, and of a narrow basal layer, lying on the myometrium and persisting after menstruation. The basal layer is a reconstruction layer. In the course of the menstrual cycle, characteristic morphological changes occur in the pars functionalis.

During the proliferative phase, between days 4 and 14 of the cycle, under the influence of estradiol, the endometrial glands increase and thicken. The tubular glands are long, and the cytogenic stroma is of very high cell density. In transverse sections, the glands present a small, plump and optically empty lumen. They are covered by dark cells that are partly cubic, partly cylindrical. Mitosis occurs both in the glands and in the stroma cells.

Between days 15 and 18 of the cycle, under the influence of progesterone, the secretory phase starts. Small basal or retronuclear vacuoles in the glands' epithelia are the first signs of secretion; they contain glycogen. In the course of the secretory phase, the endometrial glands take the tortuous shape of a cork-screw; the lumina are irregular. The epithelia have a bright cytoplasm; the cell nuclei move basally. The stroma cells are broken up and they are rather large. At the end of the secretory phase, they show a magnocellular or pseudo-decidual transformation in the area of the compacta[1]. The morphological changes of the endometrium during the secretory phase lead to a doubling of its total volume. Four days before onset of bleeding, the endometrium begins to shrink, due to decreasing activity of the corpus luteum. In cycles where conception has occurred, this shrinking fails to take place[2].

Contrary to the follicular phase, the chronological development of the endometrium during the luteal phase can be exactly dated histologically from its typical structural changes. During the first half of the luteal phase, dating is based mainly on changes of the glandular epithelium; during the second half, it is based mainly on the daily changes of the picture of the stroma[3]. At the end of the secretory phase, the bleeding begins; glandular epithelial and stromal pieces, detached from the cenobium and embedded in blood, can be discerned. Fibrin thrombi are absent. With the beginning of the menopause, senile involution of the endometrium occurs. The uterine mucosa becomes narrower, with a stroma rich in cells and fibers and with small, round glands decreasing in number[1].

Sonographic appearance of the endometrium in spontaneous cycles

The first examinations of the endometrium were performed transabdominally[4–11]. In transabdominal ultrasonography, the bladder must be filled. The sonographic thickness of the endometrium may differ according to the filling of the bladder, the angle of incidence of the ultrasound waves, the thickness of the subcutaneous fatty tissue and the feasibility of delimiting the endometrial and myometrial layers[12]. Since the improvement of vaginal ultrasound, sonographic assessment of the endometrium for functional analysis has played a more important role.

The sonographic appearance of the endometrium is based on dynamic, histological and physiological changes. Some groups[6,7,13–15] have found evidence for the fact that, both in normal and in stimulated cycles, changes in the endometrium can be detected sonographically. Bald and Hackelöer[7] divide the growth in thickness (during

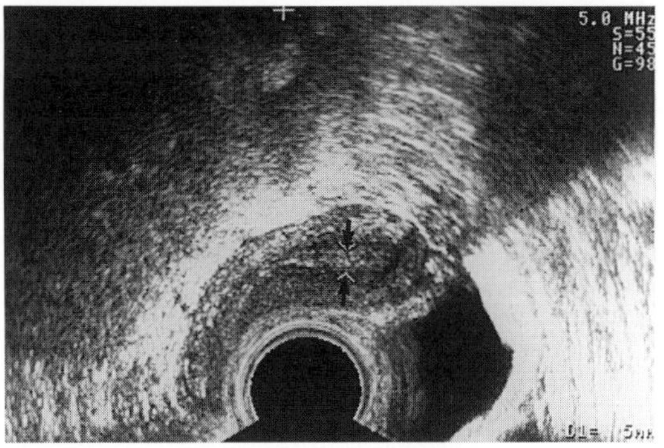

Figure 1 Endometrium in the early proliferative phase (arrows): narrow and slightly more echogenic than the surrounding endometrium

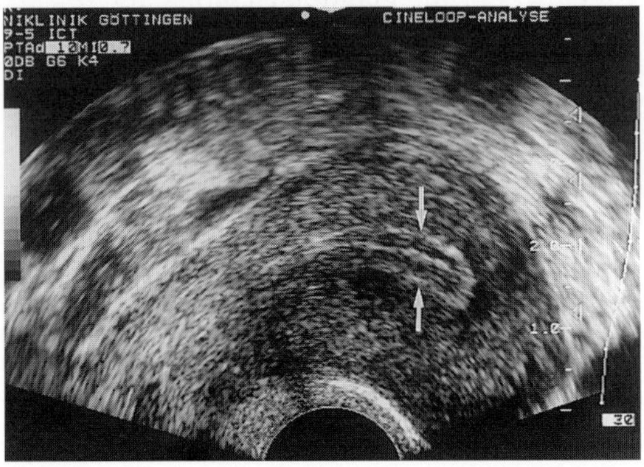

Figure 2 Late proliferative phase of the endometrium (arrows): narrow hyperreflective mid-line with a hypodense area in between

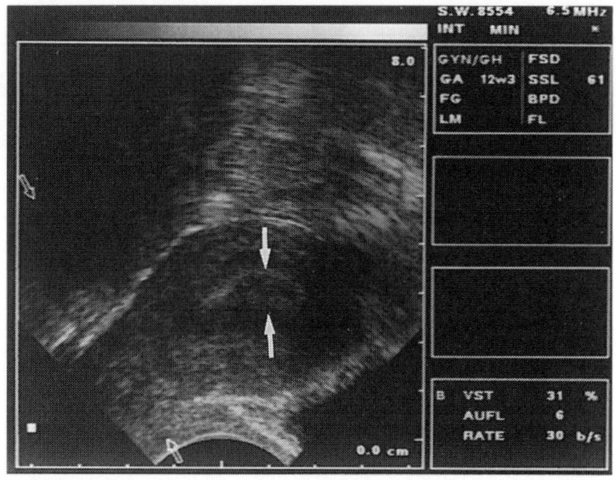

Figure 3 Endometrium in the beginning of the luteal phase (white arrows): slightly hyperechogenic halo and a distinct hypoechogenic area in between (endometrial ring sign)

the proliferative phase) into three stages and thus differentiate between six types of endometrium which again differ in their sonographic picture, whereas Deichert and Michaels[16] divide the sonographic appearance of the endometrium into four stages: proliferative type, periovulatory type and secretory types I and II.

In the early proliferative phase, the endometrium presents itself as thin and slightly more echogenic than the surrounding myometrium (Figure 1). Later on, the endometrium shows a small hyperreflective lining and a thin hyperreflective intermediate echo (Figure 2), with a hypoechogenic area lying between. The ultrasound phenomenon can be found – to a different extent – before and after ovulation. The intermediate echo corresponds to the lumen of the uterus. The exact morphological or histological structures that correlate with the echogenic lining are not known. They might correspond either to the basal layer or to the space between the endo- and the myometrium. The hypoechogenic zone between the intermediate echo and the lining corresponds to the pars functionalis and should not be confounded with the relatively hypoechogenic halo, which surrounds the basal layer towards the myometrium. The latter corresponds histologically to a vascular rete between the endometrium and the myometrium[17].

At the beginning of the luteal phase, the intermediate echo and the lining start to disappear; the endometrial picture becomes echogenic to an increasing degree. Increase of the echogenicity starts in the area of the lining and continues towards the uterine cavity; a distinct hypoechogenic area, however, can still be recognized. These changes have been described by Bald and Hackelöer[7] as 'endometrial ring sign' (Figure 3). While the rather hypoechogenic appearance of the proliferating endometrium is in accordance with its homogeneous histological structure, the conjunction of glandular and vascular changes leads to increasing echogenicity of the secretory endometrium (Figure 4). Besides these sonographic changes, Brandt and co-workers[18] have described a mild dorsal echo enchancement during the secretory phase. This phenomenon is not usually characteristic of echogenic structures; it can

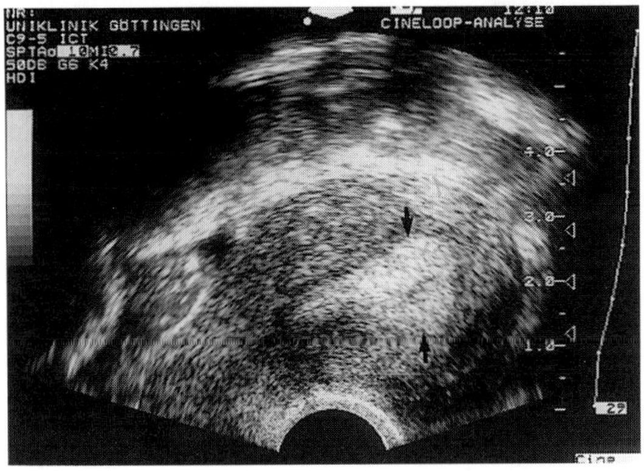

Figure 4 Late secretory phase: broad homogeneous endometrium (arrows)

rather be found in cystic cavities or cavities filled with liquid. As in hemangioma, the abundance of reflections of the secretory endometrium might be explained by the huge quantity of reflexogenic structures in the vessel walls, which have an excellent echo conduction due to the large amount of fluid. Forrest and associates[17], however, found a dorsal echo enhancement in 52% of their patients in the proliferative phase also. This indicates that this is a rather unspecific phenomenon.

In ultrasound measurements, the thickness of the endometrium first decreases during menstruation, on average from 8 to 6 mm and less. During the proliferative phase, the thickness of the endometrium increases until if reaches a periovulatory maximum. These changes run parallel with the follicular growth and the rising estradiol levels. During the luteal phase, the endometrial thickness is often still increasing. During the secretory phase, development of endometrial growth differs individually: a postovulatory decrease with subsequent increase of the thickness of the endometrium during the luteal phase, and a continuous increase going beyond the periovulatory maximum and lasting until the secretory phase may occur[16].

During the luteal phase, there is no exact correlation between the sonographically determined thickness of the endometrium and the serum progesterone or estradiol levels[10,19]. Besides the sex hormones, other parameters such as the steroid receptor ratio in the endometrium influence its development[20].

A comparison of the findings in histologically appropriate and inappropriate mucosa makes it clear that luteal development does not depend on the hormonal secretion of the corpus luteum only. It is true that the endometrial reaction is more often delayed when there is corpus luteum insufficiency, but normal function of the corpus luteum with normal progesterone levels does not necessarily lead to an appropriate development of the endometrium. The mid-luteal thickness of the endometrium in histologically appropriate mucosa with an average of 13 mm is above the level for below average endometria, 12 mm. Overlap, however, occurs rather often[16]. According to Deichert and colleagues[16], the thickness of the endometrium determined in the middle of the luteal phase should amount to 10 mm at least. Otherwise a below average mucosa has to be expected.

Corresponding with the histological changes after the menopause, the endometrium appears sonographically as a narrow, hyperechogenic line.

Sonographic findings of the endometrium prior to conception

Some groups have not found any correlation between the sonographic thickness of the endometrium during the follicular phase and the onset of a pregnancy in the same cycle[9,10,12,21–24]. However, Gonen and colleagues[25], Bergh and colleagues[26] and Cohen and colleagues[27] have postulated that the thickness of the endometrium determined by transvaginal sonography the day before puncture of the follicle or before ovulation is a predictive factor for the onset of a pregnancy. Therefore, no recommendations can be given as far as the thickness or the growth rate of the endometrium are concerned. Therefore, endometrial measurements do not allow us to break off an *in vitro* fertilization (IVF) cycle on the basis of a supposed poor chance of success.

Nor does the thickness of the endometrium in the luteal phase enable us to make a better prediction concerning the pregnancy than would be possible with laboratory diagnosis, by measurement of levels of human chorionic gonadotropin (hCG). After IVF treatment has led to conception, from day 12 after puncture of the follicle onwards, a rapid increase of the thickness of the endometrium can be observed[10]. By this time, however, serum hCG titers would be positive.

Rabinowitz and co-workers[10] proposed a minimum thickness of the endometrium of 13 mm on day 9 after puncture of the follicle; this would be the most favorable predictor of conception, as in IVF cycles, that pregnancies had occurred only under these circumstances. The type of endometrium at the time of puncture appears to have a certain predictive value; Welker and associates[22] obtained the highest number of pregnancies with the trizonal periovulatory type and no pregnancy at all with the homogeneously echogenic endometrium.

SONOGRAPHIC FINDINGS IN INFERTILE PATIENTS

Besides inadequate changes in the type of endometrium and insufficient growth rate in the course of the cycle, the following findings can be detected more often in infertile patients: endometrial polyps, intracavitary myoma, submucous myoma and intracavitary fluid pools as a result of cervical stenosis; the latter have to be explored operatively.

Patients with luteal phase deficiency

An abnormal appearance of the endometrium may indicate an ovarian dysfunction[28]. If luteal function and endometrial reaction are normal, a secretory type of endometrium with a thickness of > 10 mm is to be expected during the luteal phase. Patients with appropriate endometrial histology usually comply with these criteria[16]. Orientating functional diagnostics of the luteal phase or of the endometrium factor can be carried out by means of vaginosonographic assessment of the endometrial type and of the thickness of the endometrium on day 7 ± 1 postovulation[16] If, in a spontaneous or stimulated cycle, there is evidence of a conspicuous, i.e. not appropriate, type of endometrium, or if the thickness of the endometrium is below 10 mm, histological diagnosis of the endometrium can be obtained in the same cycle.

Patients with polycystic ovarian disease

The thickness of the endometrium seems to be a function of the duration of the estrogen effect rather than a function of the plasma estrogen levels. Thus, endometrial hyperplasia in patients with polycystic ovarian disease appears to be a consequence of the elevated estrogen levels due to the insufficient ovarian–hypophyseal/hypothalamic feedback mechanism[21].

Patients with hyperprolactinemia

Hyperprolactinemic patienst present a thin, rather echogenic endometrium both in the proliferative and in the secretory phase[27].

Sonographic endometrial findings in stimulated cycles

Both in spontaneous cycles and in IVF cycles overstimulated with gonadotropin/clomiphene, the growth rate of the endometrium and the sonomorphology are about the same during the whole cycle, in spite of serum estrogen levels differing significantly[12,29–31]. According to Randall and colleagues[31], the thickness of the endometrium in treated and in non-treated cycles on average does not differ very much or does not differ at all at corresponding moments. Giorlandino and colleagues[19] and Shoham and associates[32] reported that in stimulated cycles there is a positive correlation between the estradiol level and the thickness of the endometrium. According to Rabinowitz and co-workers[10], Welcker and co-workers[33] and Sterzig and co-workers[24], neither the ultrasound grading nor the histology are associated with the serum estradiol or progesterone levels. This contrasts with non-stimulated cycles where a close correlation was found[28,34].

Stimulation with clomiphene alone leads to significantly thinner endometria due to the anti-estrogenic effect of clomiphene[27,30].

In a comparison between different stimulation schedules in IVF cycles with regard to thickness of the endometrium, the combination of clomiphene and human menopausal gonadotropin (hMG) seems to have a significantly poorer effect on endometrial growth than do analogs of gonadotropin releasing hormone (GnRH)[35].

Sonographic findings in stimulated cycles of patients with hypogonadotropic hypogonadism

Induction of ovulation with follicle stimulating hormone (FSH) or hMG in patients with hypogonadotropic hypogonadism leads to proliferation of the endometrium, which can be viewed by transvaginal sonography as a result of the growth in length. Shoham and colleagues[36] reported that the endometrium was significantly thicker in patients treated with hMG than in those treated with FSH.

Endometrial findings after suppression therapy

The effects of a treatment with GnRH analogs for down-regulation of hypophyseal pulsatility of luteinizing hormone (LH) can be visualized sonographically. Thus a thickened endometrium ($\geq$8 mm) of the secretory type may indicate that therapy was too short or insufficient. A hypoechogenic, thin endometrium (<8 mm) may give evidence of the achieved hormonal suppression.

SONOGRAPHIC DEPICTION OF INTRAUTERINE DEVICES

After ovulation inhibitors, the intrauterine device (IUD) is the second most effective contraceptive method, and is non-invasive. Pregnancies may occur after an undetected IUD expulsion, after dislocation of the IUD and after incorrect placement of the IUD. The failure rate (pregnancy) is 0.5–5 unwanted pregnancies per 1200 months of application or per 100 woman-years[37]. Bernaschek and associates[38] and Meyenburg[39] were able to show that, in 80% of those cases of unwanted pregnancy with an IUD, the device had been placed too low. Contraceptive effectiveness depends on the type of device, the time of use, the correct placement and the anatomy of the woman. Therefore, changes of position and form of the uterus, such as sinistro- or dextroposition, retroflexio uteri fixata or a steep anteflexion, or

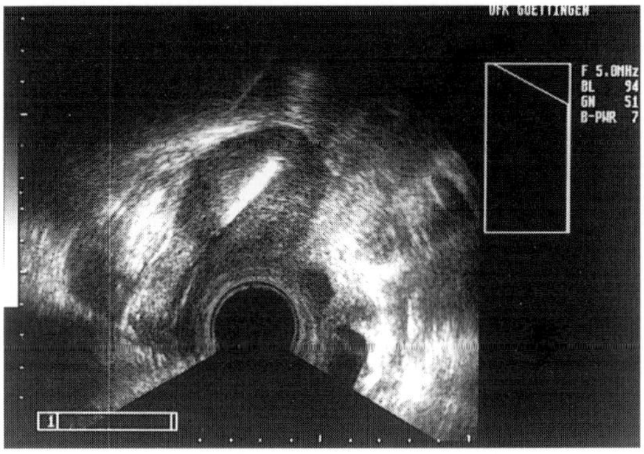

Figure 5 Correctly placed intrauterine device

changes of growth, such as myohyperplasia, may impair the correct placement. If there are submucous myoma or intracavitary polyps, it may even be impossible to insert the IUD. Whereas in the past control of the IUD was only through the checking of the IUD strings and nothing could be said about the exact intrauterine localization of the device, nowadays control of the IUD's position can easily be carried out by means of ultrasound[37,40–44] (Figure 5).

Currently, different types of IUD are available: plastic IUDs (Lippes-Loop®), IUDs containing copper (Copper-T®, Copper-7®, Multiload®) and IUDs containing progesterone (Progestasert-Pessar®). Depending on the type of IUD and provided it is placed correctly in the cavity, the device can be visualized sonographically in the longitudinal section as an echogenic stripe (Copper-T) or as five echogenic points (Lippes-Loop). In the transverse section, the Copper-T presents itself as a hyperechogenic point in the middle of the corpus; in the area of the fundus, the arms of the device, which present themselves as a hyperechogenic horizontal line, can be seen, provided that unfolding has occurred. The Multiload shows three echogenic points lying beside one another.

The sonographically measurable distance between the fundus uteri and the end of the device lying close to the fundus is important, in order to assess whether or not the IUD is in place. By rule of thumb, this distance should not be smaller than 2 cm[41]. With this measurement, however, the thickness of the uterine wall, which differs individually, is not taken into account. Bernaschek and associates[40] therefore gave a formula, taking into account the thickness of the anterior and posterior wall of the uterus. According to this formula, the position of the device is correct if the distance between the fundus and the upper end of the IUD does not amount to more than four-thirds of the average thickness of the uterine wall: [(anterior wall + posterior wall)12] × 1.33. In addition, care should be taken that the arms of the device are properly unfolded. This enables assessment of the length of the device in the longitudinal section, and also assessment of the arms of the device in the transverse section.

Besides the fundus–IUD distance, the distance between the upper end of the device and the base of the endometrium seems to be a practical measurement for assessment of the correct position in hyperplastic uteri. This distance should not exceed 5 mm.

Bernaschek and colleagues[40] and Meyenburg and co-workers[42] reported that, in 10% and 16%, respectively, of all women with an IUD, the device was not in the right place. In these cases, the device should be removed, as it may impair contraceptive effectiveness, and also cause pain in the lower abdomen and bleeding. The position of the IUD ought to be controlled sonographically immediately after 4 and 12 weeks' time, as dislocation or expulsion of the device occurs mainly within the first months after insertion[45].

If a woman becomes pregnant with an IUD in place, the risk of spontaneous abortion is 50% compared with that in normal pregnancies. If the IUD is removed early, the risk of spontaneous abortion decreases to 20–25%[46]. Besides the elevated abortion rate, there is an increased risk of premature birth and still birth. After removal of the IUD within the first trimester, the abortion rate can be decreased by a factor of four; beyond the first trimester, however, only by a factor of two. The premature birth rate decreases by a factor of five, and the stillbirth rate by a factor of two after removal of the IUD[47].

The abortion risk after extraction can be pre-estimated by sonographic localization of the IUD with regard to its proximity to the embryo. While a cervically dislocated IUD in general can be removed easily, an IUD located cranial to the embryo should remain *in situ*.

Recommendation for the removal of an IUD in a pregnant woman has nothing to do, however, with a recommendation or an indication for interruption of pregnancy. There is no reason for such a procedure, particularly as there is no evidence at all of the teratogenicity of IUDs[48].

References

1. Sandritter, T. C. (1983). *Histopathologie. Lehrbuch und Atlas*, Vol. 9, p. 219. (Stuttgart, New York: Schattenhauer-Verlag)
2. Dallenbach-Hellweg, G. (1988). The endometrium in natural and artificial luteal phases. *Hum. Reprod.*, **2**, 165–8
3. Dallenbach-Hellweg, G. (1981). *Endometrium*, Vol. 2, pp. 49–82. (Berlin, Heidelberg, New York: Springer)
4. Hall, D. A., Hann, L. E., Ferrucci, J. T., Black, E. B., Braitman, B. S., Crowley, W. F., Nikrui, N. and Kelley, J. A. (1979). Sonographic morphology of the normal menstrual cycle. *Radiology*, **133**, 185
5. Christie, A. D. (1981). Ultrasound and infertility – fundamentals. In Christie, A. D. (ed.) *Ultrasound and Infertility*, pp. 1–14. (Old Ochard, USA: Chartwell Bratt)
6. Sakamoto, C. and Nakano, H., (1982). The echogenic endometrium and alterations during menstrual cycle. *Int. J. Gynaecol. Obstet.*, **20**, 255–9
7. Bald, R. and Hackelöer, B. J. (1983). Ultraschalldarstellung verschiedener Endometriumformen. In Otto, R. and Jan, F. X. (eds.) *Ultraschalldiagnostik 1982*, p. 187. (Stuttgart: Thieme)
8. Fleischer, A. C., Pittaway, D., Beard, L., Thieme, G., Bundy, A., James, A. and Wentz, A. (1984). Sonographic depiction of endometrial changes occurring with ovulation induction. *J. Ultrasound Med.*, **3**, 344
9. Glissant, A., de Mouzon, J. and Frydman, R. (1985). Ultrasound study of the endometrium during *in vitro* fertilization cycles. *Fertil. Steril.*, **44**, 786–90
10. Rabinowitz, R., Laufer, N., Lewin, A., Navot, D., Bar, I., Margalioth, E. and Schenker, J. J. G. (1986). The value of ultrasonographic endometrial

measurement in the prediction of pregnancy following *in vitro* fertilization. *Fertil. Steril.*, **45**, 824–8
11. Deichert, U., Hackelöer, B. J. and Daume, E. (1986). The sonographic and endocrinologic evaluation of the endometrium in the luteal phase. *Hum. Reprod.*, **1**, 219–22
12. Fleischer, A. C., Kalemeris, G. C. and Entman, S. S. (1986). Sonographic depiction of the endometrium during normal cycles. *Ultrasound Med. Biol.*, **12**, 271–7
13. Bald, R. and Hackelöer, B. J. (1982). Neue sonographische Kriterien zur Darstellung der stattgehabten Ovulation. In Kratochwil, A. E. (ed.) *Reinold: Ultraschalldiagnostik 81*, p. 224. (Stuttgart: Thieme)
14. Merz, E., Schaller, C., Hoffmann, G. and Pollow, K. (1985). Ultrasonic evidence of endometrium in correlation to the follicular development and the hormonal parameters in patients stimulated with clomiphene citrate. *Vortrag XI. Weltkongreß Gynäkologie u. Geburtshilfe*, Berlin
15. Nakano, H., Sakamoto, C., Koyangi, T. and Kubota, S. (1982). Endometrial images by ultrasound. *Acta Obstet. Gynecol Jpn.*, **34**, 275
16. Deichert, U. and Michaels, W. (1993). Zyklische Veränderungen am Uterus. In Deichert, U., Duda, V. and Schlief, R. (eds.) *Funktionelle Sonographie in Gynäkologie und Reproduktionsmedizin*. (Berlin: Springer-Verlag)
17. Forrest, T. S., Elyaderani, M. K., Muilenburg, M. I., Bewtra, C., Kable, W. T. and Sullivan, P. (1988). Cyclic endometrial changes: US assessment with histologic correlation. *Radiology*, **167**, 233–7
18. Brandt, T. D., Levy, E. B., Grant, T. H., Marut, E. and Leland, J. (1985). Endometrial echo and its significance in female infertility. *Radiology*, **137**, 225–9
19. Giorlandino, C., Gleicher, N., Nanni, C., Vizzone, A., Gentili, P. and Taramanni, C. (1987). The sonographic picture of endometrium in spontaneous and induced cycles. *Fertil. Steril.*, **47**, 508–11
20. Wentz, A. C. (1979). Physiologic and clinical considerations in luteal phase defects. *Clin. Obstet. Gynaecol.*, **22**, 169
21. Adams, J. M., Tan, S. L., Wheeler, M. J., Morris, D. V., Jacobs, H. S. and Franks, S. (1988). Uterine growth in the follicular phase of spontaneous ovulatory cycles and during luteinizing hormone-releasing hormone-induced cycles in women with normal or polycystic ovaries. *Fertil. Steril.*, **49**, 52–5
22. Welker, B., Gembruch, U., Diedrich, K. and Krebs, D. (1988). Endosonography of the endometrium with respect of IVF outcome. *Hum. Reprod.*, **3** (Suppl. I), 42
23. Thickman, D., Arger, P., Tureck, R., Blasco, L., Mintz, M. and Coleman, B. (1986). Sonographic assessment of the endometrium in patients undergoing *in vitro* fertilization. *J. Ultrasound Med.*, **5**, 197–201
24. Sterzig, K., Grab, D., Rosenbusch, B., Hamers, G. and Dallenbach-Hellweg, G. (1991). Zur Rezeptivität des Endometriums: Vergleich sonographischer und histologischer Befunde nach hormoneller Stimulation. *Geburtshilf. Frauenheilk.*, **51**, 554–8
25. Gonen, Y., Casper, R. F., Jacobson, W. and Blankier, J. (1989). Endometrial thickness and growth during ovarian stimulation: a possible predictor of implantation in *in vitro* fertilization. *Fertil. Steril.*, **52**, 446–50
26. Bergh, C., Hillensjö, T. and Nilsson, L. (1992). Sonographic evaluation of the endometrium in *in vitro* fertilization IVF cycles. *Acta Obstet. Gynecol. Scand.*, **71**, 624–8
27. Cohen, B. M., Berry, L., Roethemeyer, V. and Smith, D. (1992). Sonographic assessment of late proliferative phase endometrium during ovulation induction. *J. Reprod. Med.*, **37**, 685–90
28. Yoshimitsu, K., Nakamura, G. and Nakano, H. (1989). Dating sonographic endometrial images in the normal ovulatory cycle. *Int. J. Gynaecol. Obstet.*, **28**, 33–9
29. Sakamoto, C., Yoshimitsu, K., Nakamura, G., Ootsuka, H. and Yoshida, K. (1988). Sonographic study of the endometrial responses to ovarian hormones in patients receiving ovarian stimulation. *Int. J. Gynaecol. Obstet.*, **27**, 407–14
30. Imoedemhe, D. A. G., Shaw, R. W., Kirkland, A. and Chan, R. (1987). Ultrasound measurement of endometrial thickness on different ovarian stimulation regimes during *in-vitro* fertilization. *Hum. Reprod.*, **2**, 545–7
31. Randall, J. M., Fisk, N. M., McTavish, A. and Templeton, A. A. (1989). Transvaginal ultrasonic assessment of endometrial growth in spontaneous and hyperstimulated menstrual cycles. *Br. J. Obstet. Gynaecol.*, **96**, 954–9
32. Shoham, Z., Di Carlo, C., Patel, A., Conway, G. S. and Jacobs, H. S. (1991). Is it possible to run a successful ovulation induction program based solely on ultrasound monitoring? The importance of endometrial measurements. *Fertil. Steril.*, **56**, 836–41
33. Welker, B. G., Gembruch, U., Diedrich, K., Al-Hasani, S. and Krebs, D. (1989). Transvaginal sonography of the endometrium during ovum pickup in stimulated cycles for *in vitro* fertilization. *J. Ultrasound Med.*, **8**, 549–53
34. Hackelöer, B. J. (1984). Ultrasound scanning of the ovarian cycle. *J. In Vitro Fertil. Embryo Transfer*, **1**, 217
35. Rogers, P. A. W., Polson, D., Murphy, C. R., Hosie, M., Susil, B. and Leoni, M. (1991). Correlation of endometrial histology, morphometry, and ultrasound appearance after different stimulation protocols. *Fertil. Steril.*, **55**, 583–7
36. Shoham, Z., Balen, A., Patel, A. and Jacobs, H. S.

(1991). Results of ovulation induction using human menopausal gonadotropin or purified follicle-stimulating hormone in hypogonadotropic hypogonadism patients. *Fertil. Steril.*, **56**, 1048–53
37. Cochrane, W. J. (1984). Ultrasonography and the intrauterine device. In Steel, W. B. and Cochrane W. J. (eds.) *Gynecologic Ultrasound.* (New York: Churchill Livingstone)
38. Bernaschek, G., Spernol, R. and Beck, A. (1981). IUD-Lage bei intrauterinen Schwangerschaften. *Geburtshilf. Frauenheilk.*, **41**, 645
39. Meyenburg, H. (1978). Anwendung der Ultraschall-Schnittbildtechnik zur Darstellung von Intrauterinspiralen. *Geburtshilf. Frauenheilk.*, **38**, 950
40. Bernaschek, G., Endler, M. and Beck, A. (1981). Zur Lagekontrolle von Intrauterinpessaren. *Geburtshilf. Frauenheilk.*, **41**, 556
41. Hansmann, M., Hackelöer, B. and Staudach, J. (1985). *Ultraschalldiagnostik in Geburtshilfe und Gynäkologie.* (Berlin: Springer)
42. Meyenburg, M., Höbich, D. and Hein, H. W. (1981). Sonographische Darstellung von Cu-T-Intrauterinpessaren. *Ultraschall*, **2**, 153
43. Nelson, L. H. and Miller, J. B. (1979). Real-time ultrasound in locating intrauterine contraceptive devices. *Obstet. Gynecol.*, **54**, 711
44. Nemes, G. and Kerenyi, T. D. (1971). Ultrasonic localization of the IUCD: a new technique. *Am. J. Obstet. Gynecol.*, **109**, 12–19
45. Schmidt, E. H., Wagner, H., Quakernack, K. and Beller, F. K. (1979). Ergebnisse der Lageüberwachung von Intrauterinpessaren durch Ultraschall. *Geburtshilf. Frauenheilk.*, **39**, 138
46. Tauber, P. F. and Nohlen, M. (1984). Alternative IUP. In Breckwoldt, M. (ed.) *Empfängnisverhütung – Bewertung verschiedener Methoden aus heutiger Sicht. Med Wiss Buchreihe*, pp. 35–43. (Berlin: Schering AG)
47. Krieglsteiner, P. (1984). Zur Vermeidung von MP-Komplikationen. In Breckwoldt, M. (ed.) *Empfängnisverhütung – Bewertung verschiedener Methoden aus heutiger Sicht. Med Wiss Buchreihe*, pp. 45–51. (Berlin: Schering AG)
48. Schweppe, K.-W. (1983). Das Mißbildungsrisiko bei Gravidität trotz liegenden Intrauterinpessars ist nicht erhöht. *Gyne*, **4**, 7–8

Pathological findings of the postmenopausal endometrium

5

R. Osmers, J. Puchta and A. Suren

The introduction of vaginosonography into clinical practice in 1986 has added an extra dimension to the visualization of the woman's internal genital tract. Besides the ovaries, uterine structures are now accessible to assessment, which before had only been possible by invasive methods.

SONOGRAPHIC FEATURES OF ENDOMETRIAL INFLAMMATORY DISEASES

If there are inflammatory changes in the endometrium, they present both in the pre- and in the postmenopause as a typically widened and echogenic endometrium. The picture corresponds with the late secretory phase. We have seen cases of chronic endometritis in the postmenopause that show an endometrial thickness of 22 mm. In rare cases, such inflammatory changes can be associated with secretions into the uterine cavity in the form of a sero- or pyometra; however, the latter generally corresponds with more reflexogenic fluid pools in the uterine cavity. These cannot be distinguished from a hematometra. In such a case, the endometrium may take quite an irregular, bizarre shape towards the uterine cavity, so that resemblance to an endometrial carcinoma may be striking (Figure 1). The boundary between the endometrium and the myometrium is often poorly outlined, frequently having the consequence that – especially with an unexperienced examiner – the prima vista diagnosis of an endometrial carcinoma is established. In distinct endomyometritis the echogenicity of the myometrium is somewhat increased, compared to that of a uterus without inflammatory changes.

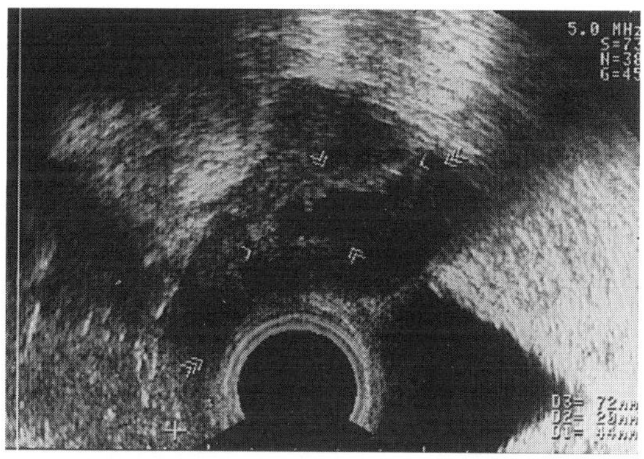

Figure 1 Anteflexed uterus with irregularly shaped endometrium and small pyometra. Histology: endometritis

SONOGRAPHIC FEATURES IN PREMENOPAUSAL WOMEN WITH ATYPICAL BLEEDING

In atypical bleeding in the premenopause, besides clinical and cytological examination, assessment should be made of the ovaries and the cervix uteri (as has already been mentioned in Chapter 2). In bleeding disorders, the most frequent pathological benign changes of the uterine cavity that can be visualized sonographically are polyps and submucous myoma (Figures 2 and 3). Large intramural myomas with impression of the uterine cavity can be another cause of bleeding.

Differentiation between submucous myomas and polyps can be difficult. Both are characterized sonographically by an echogenic reflection pattern. Principally, the polyp grows towards the uterine cavity only, so that in the case of echogenic tumors, which grow both towards the uterine cavity and towards the myometrium, submucous

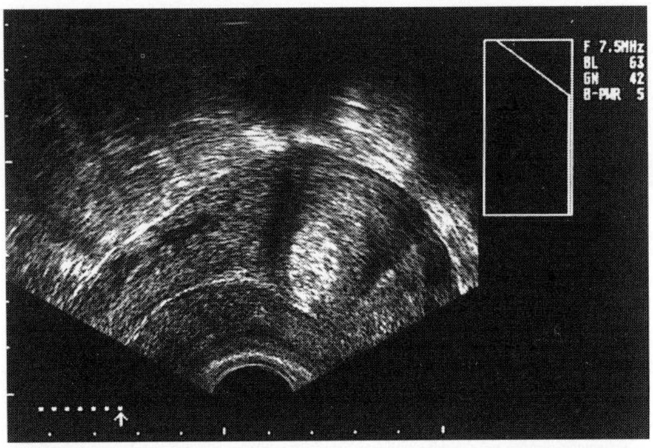

Figure 2 Anteflexed uterus with hyperechogenic submucous myoma protruding into the uterine cavity. Histology: submucous myoma

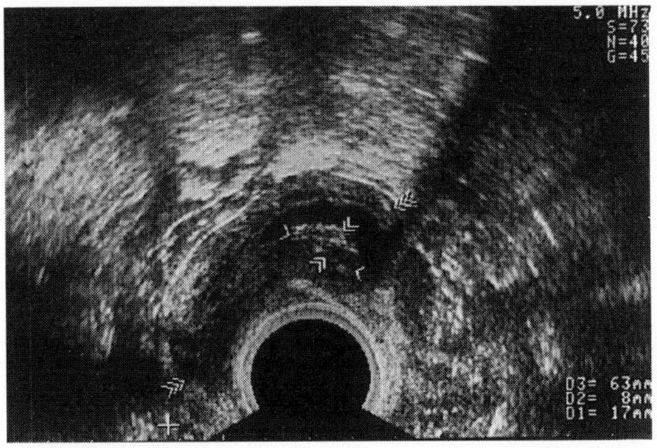

Figure 4 Depiction of a small polyp located at the uterine wall after fluid instillation into the uterine cavity. Histology: fibrous polyp

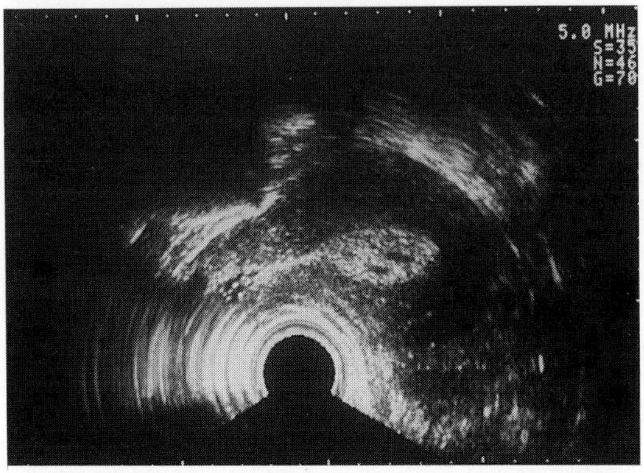

Figure 3 Anteflexed uterus showing a thickened, hyperechogenic endometrium with small inclusion cysts. Histology: cystic polyp with small areas of adenomatous hyperplasia without atypia

myoma can be assumed. In many cases, differentiation between a polyp and a myoma is easier after instillation of saline solution into the uterine cavity (see Chapter 6). In addition, this may facilitate assignment of the wall to which the polyp is attached (Figure 4). It must be stressed, however, that in some cases a final differentiation can be established by hysteroscopy or histology only.

SONOGRAPHIC FEATURES OF THE ENDOMETRIUM IN AMENORRHEA

The sonographic picture of the uterus of amenorrheic patients with estrogen deficiency corresponds with the picture of the postmenopausal uterus, showing a thin endometrial lining of less than 2 mm (Figure 5). In the case of secondary amenorrhea, with an endometrium corresponding with the late secretory phase, one has to be aware of a persistent follicle or of an ongoing pregnancy (Figure 6). In Asherman syndrome, vaginosonography is not very useful. The sonographic pictures often correspond with those of a narrow endometrium during the secretory phase, but filling up of the uterine cavity and the subsequent missing distension of the uterine cavity may contribute to the differential diagnosis.

SONOGRAPHIC FEATURES OF THE POSTMENOPAUSAL ENDOMETRIUM

Normal sonographic depiction

Although cytology serves well as a screening method for cervical cancer, it must be accepted that the cervical smear is not the right method for early detection of endometrial carcinoma. Between 1980 and 1990 at the University and Medical School (Department of Obstetrics and Gynecology) of Göttingen, in 17 293 postmenopausal patients only one asymptomatic endometrial carcinoma was detected by means of cervical cytology. This emphasizes the subordinate role of cytology for detection of endometrial carcinoma and its preliminary stages. In view of these difficulties, numerous instruments have been

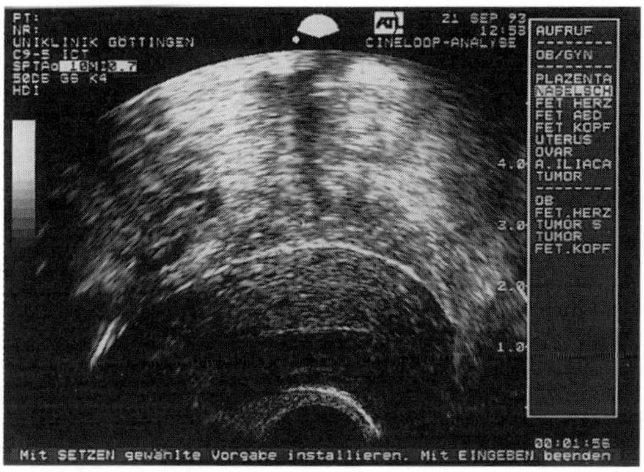

Figure 5 Anteflexed uterus with a thin endometrium in a patient with secondary amenorrhea

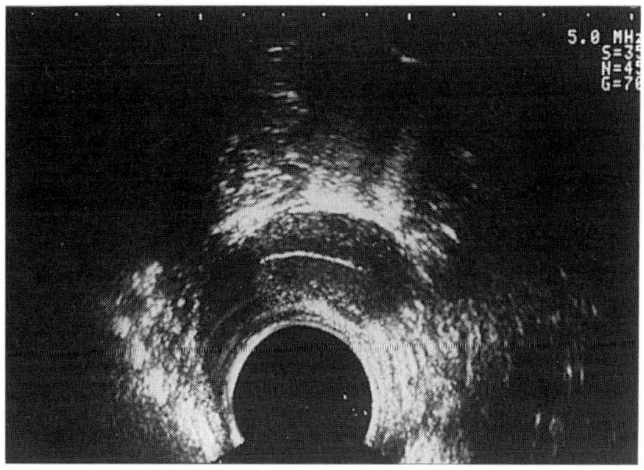

Figure 7 Typical linear echogenic endometrium of a postmenopausal uterus

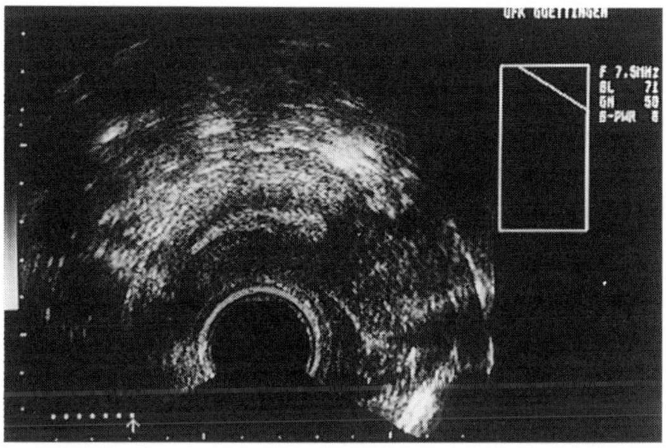

Figure 6 Anteflexed uterus with a thickened endometrium in a patient with secondary amenorrhea due to a persisting follicle

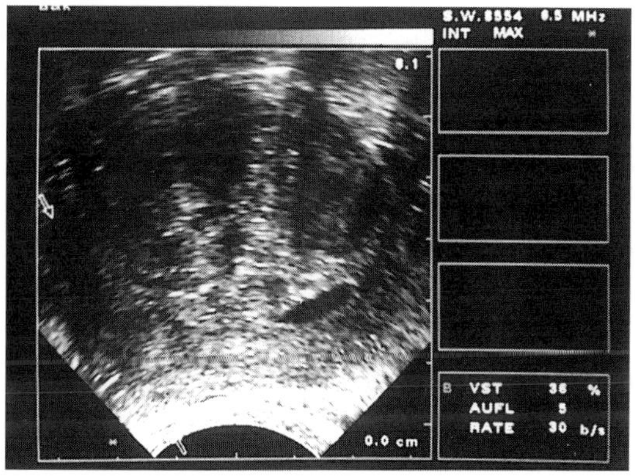

Figure 8 Postmenopausal uterus with a large fibrous myoma in the posterior uterine wall. The thin atrophic endometrium is difficult to identify (arrow), but it surrounds the small serometra adjacent to the myoma

developed in order to obtain material from the uterine cavity. This method of examination, however, comes up against limiting factors, such as difficulties of interpretation of the findings, the necessity of painful dilatation, little acceptance on the part of the patients and time-consuming procedures; all these disadvantages make it an inappropriate technique.

Vaginosonographic examination, however, has become an examination technique that is accepted by postmenopausal women in particular, and which gives the less experienced examiner an overall view of the internal genital tract in the female.

Sonographically, the endometrium in the postmenopause corresponds with that in the early follicular phase[1–5]. It appears as a small, linear, echogenic structure[6] (Figure 7), which corresponds with the stratum basale[7,8]. From histomorphological examinations, it is known that the postmenopausal endometrial thickness (single layer of the endometrium) amounts to 0.5 mm and very rarely (even in cystic atrophic endometrium) exceeds 3 mm[9–11]. In nearly all cases the endometrium can be visualized sonographically. Difficulties might arise from intracervical myoma or large uteri myomatosi (Figure 8). In a survey of sonographically examined postmenopausal endometria dating from 1965, in only 0.4% had visualization of the endometrium not been possible at all[12–20]. These results correspond well with the early works of Coleman and associates, who were able to visualize the endometrium by means of transabdominal sonography in only 27%, whereas vaginosonographically, they succeeded in 100%[21]. The first publications on the possibility of early detection of endometrial carcinoma through measurement of the thickness of the endometrium date from 1987[22].

Contrary to early methods of measurement of the thickness of the endometrium, today – according to general agreement – measurement should be carried out as follows: the uterus is viewed vaginosonographically in the longitudinal section and the total thickness of the endometrium is measured in the largest diameter. In the case of a serometra, mucometra or hematometra, the thickness of the fluid pool in the uterine cavity is subtracted from the total thickness.

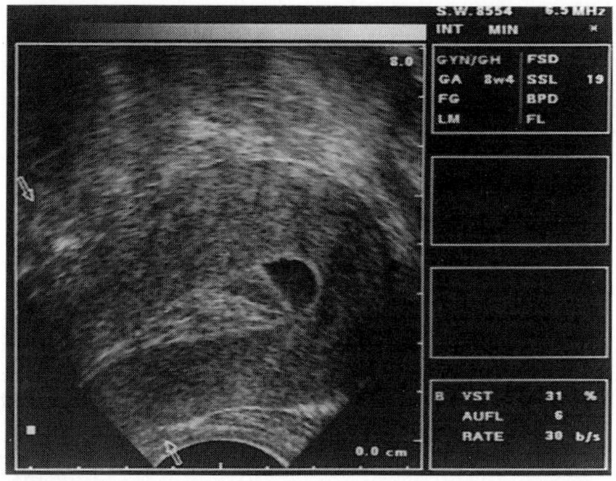

Figure 9 Postmenopausal patient with atypical bleeding: thin echogenic endometrium and distended uterine cavity by a hematometra and small clottings. Histology: atrophic endometrium

Sonographic findings with atypical bleeding

The normal endometrial picture in the postmenopause is that of an echogenic endometrial lining. In patients with postmenopausal bleeding, the endometria are considerably thicker than in asymptomatic women[33]. In a published survey of 1052 vaginosonographic examinations in patients with postmenopausal bleeding, 12.5% on average had endometrial carcinoma[12–20,24]. In none of the cases was endometrial carcinoma found when the thickness of the endometrium was below 5 mm (Figure 9). In our own examinations of 233 patients with postmenopausal bleeding, with a chosen cut-off level of 8 mm, endometrial carcinoma could not be detected either. Endometrial thickness above 8 mm, however, was associated with endometrial carcinoma in 21%. This chosen cut-off level applies not only to carcinoma, but also to its preliminary stages, such as adenomatous hyperplasia with atypia. In our population of women with postmenopausal bleeding, 6% of cases of adenomatous hyperplasia (Figure 10) were confirmed histologically with thickness of the endometrium exceeding 8 mm, but none at all with thickness remaining below 8 mm. This agrees with the results of other authors as far as the cut-off level of 5 mm is concerned.

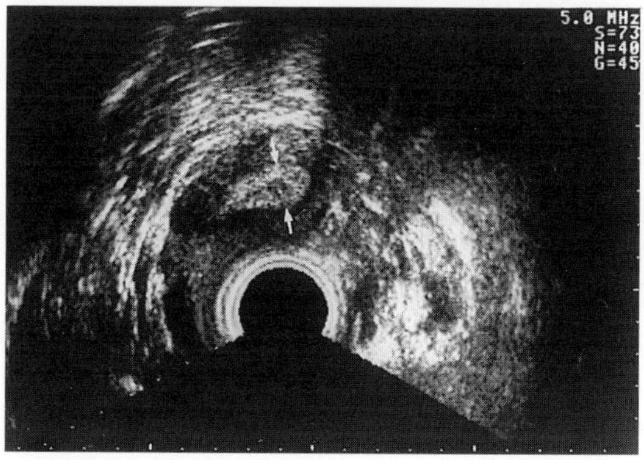

Figure 10 Anteflexed uterus with thickened postmenopausal endometrium (arrow). Histology: adenomatous hyperplasia without atypia

At first sight, this might lead to the conclusion that, with an endometrium measuring less than 5 mm in the vaginosonographic picture, one is on the safe side. It must be emphasized, however, that due to the biological behavior of carcinoma they may occur – at least in isolated cases – just as well with endometria measuring less than 5 mm; this is probably only a question of correspondingly large numbers of cases. It is up to future studies to clarify how far, in patients with endometrial thickness below 5 mm and postmenopausal bleeding, dilatation and curettage might be avoidable under certain circumstances with the help of sonographic follow-up[17].

With regard to the chosen cut-off level, differ-

Table 1 Literature review of 2670 cases investigated by transvaginosonography and clarified histologically by dilation and curettage in postmenopausal women with atypical bleeding. Sensitivity, specificity, positive and negative predictive values and cut-off levels are given

Authors	*n*	*Sensitivity* (%)	*Specificity* (%)	*Positive predictive value* (%)	*Negative predictive value* (%)	*Cut-off level* (mm)
Abu-Hmeidan *et al.*[16]	120	87.1	83.3	82.0	88.0	10
Brandner *et al.*[68]	221	93.0	96.0	79.0	96.0	6
Dorum *et al.*[18]	100	80.0	60.0	26.0	94.4	5
Granberg *et al.*[17]	205	100	96.0	87.3	—	8
Granberg *et al.*[69]	1160	96.7	67.0	59.9	97.6	5
Karlsson *et al.*[19]	105	97.0	81.0	72.0	98.0	5
Osmers *et al.*[20]	233	100	69.4	20.8	100	8
Schweighart *et al.*[70]	113	76.0	45.5	15.6	93.8	8
Seelbach-Göbel *et al.*[71]	232	94.9	43.5	25.3	97.7	8
Smith *et al.*[24]	96	100	61.0	39.0	100	8
Varner *et al.*[14]	15	96.7	100	100	90	4
Weigel *et al.*[15]	70	100	98.2	98.4	100	7
Total	2670	93.5	75.1	50.6	96.0	4–10

ent sensitivities and specificities for the detection of endometrial carcinoma by means of vaginosonography were achieved (Table 1). In 2670 evaluated examinations of patients with endometrial carcinoma, cut-off levels between 4 and 10 mm were chosen. The average sensitivity of the examination technique was 93.5%, the specificity 75.1%, the positive predictive value 50.6% and the negative predictive value 96.0% (Figure 11). The importance of vaginosonography on the one hand lies in the determination of patients at risk for endometrial carcinoma and on the other hand lies in the exclusion of atrophic, normal findings.

Attempts to use, besides the measurement of the endometrial thickness, morphological criteria for the assessment of the endometrium have so far not gained acceptance, as the majority of the sonomorphological criteria were barely reproducible or were not reproducible at all.

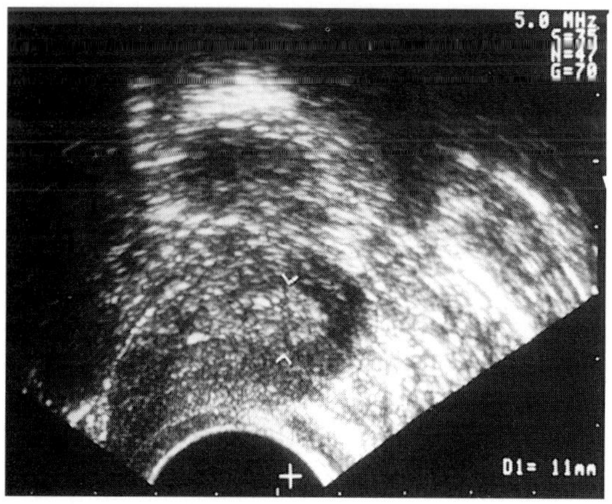

Figure 11 Anteflexed uterus with 11-mm thick endometrium in a postmenopausal woman. Histology: well-differentiated adenocarcinoma of the endometrium stage Ia (FIGO)

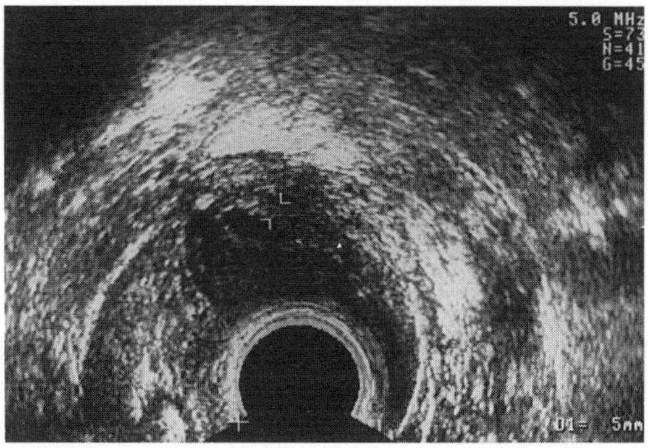

Figure 12 Retroflexed uterus with a small serometra and 5-mm thick endometrium (single layer; corresponds to 10 mm double layer) in an asymptomatic woman. Histology: well-differentiated endometrial cancer stage Ia (FIGO)

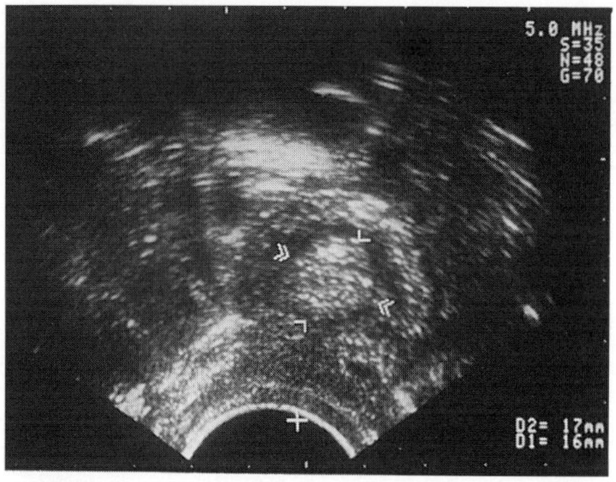

Figure 13 Well-confined echogenic tumor of the uterine cavity. Histology: endometrial cancer, stage Ib (FIGO)

Pathological sonographic findings in asymptomatic postmenopausal women

In many industrialized countries, endometrial carcinoma has advanced to being the most common genital neoplasia in women. Postmenopausal bleeding is the presenting early symptom in 80–90% of cases of endometrial carcinoma, as screening methods for early detection of endometrial carcinoma have not proven appropriate. Although endometrial carcinoma has a relatively high overall 5-year survival rate in comparison with cervical cancer and ovarian cancer, patients with invasion of the tumor into the outer third of the myometrium are at risk of metastasis into the pelvic lymph nodes in 46% of cases and into the paraortic lymph nodes in 29% of cases[25]. Therefore, early diagnosis of endometrial carcinoma is of crucial clinical importance.

Of all cases, 75–80% are diagnosed after the menopause[26]; the age peak at diagnosis is 55–65 years[11,27].

Of patients in the postmenopause, 90.2% have an endometrial thickness below 8 mm[28–30]. Of 1139 patients who had been screened vaginosonographically and who had endometrial thickness above 8 mm, 3.5% had endometrial carcinoma[14,20,29–31] (Figure 12). Sensitivity and specificity in asymptomatic patients do not differ from those who have postmenopausal bleeding. The histological results are almost identical in both groups and independent of the clinical picture[23]. It must be emphasized, however, that these values refer to postmenopausal women without hormonal replacement therapy. Therefore, one has to ensure that patients meet the requirements of more than 2 years of amenorrhea, in order to avoid too many proliferative endometria with false-positive results. In addition, hormones for replacement therapy should not have been administered within the last 6 months. When interpreting the current results, one has to take into account that the number of correctly detected endometrial carcinomas goes hand in hand with a high rate of benign findings. Measurement of the endometrial thickness only enables us to detect a population at risk, where endometrial carcinoma is more frequent. Up to the present time, the endometrial carcinoma itself is not accessible to sonomorphological methods of assessment and cannot be distinguished – at least at a preliminary stage – from benign endometrial changes (Figure 13).

The sonographic examiner must realize that the application of a cut-off level represents in any case a compromise between the chosen specificity and sensitivity. If, as in the chosen example, a cut-off level of 8 mm is chosen, 9.8% of sonographically suspicious findings in the postmenopause must be expected. Nevertheless, 2.2% of all endometrial carcinomas will be overlooked as a result of a cut-off level of 8 mm. A cut-off level of

5 mm would be an increase of safety as far as detection of endometrial carcinoma is concerned, but would be linked with a higher rate of operative intervention. When the number of benign pathological findings is reduced by the choice of a cut-off level of 12 mm, the number of necessary operations may be reduced to 5.4%, but the number of undetected carcinomas in turn will rise from 2.2 to 4.6%. It remains to be seen how far adjuvant sonographic examination techniques such as color Doppler might be able to contribute to a better discrimination.

This is why, for postmenopausal patients without hormonal replacement therapy, we suggest the following clinical procedure:

(1) Endometrial thickness up to 5 mm is interpreted as a normal finding; the next examination should be carried out in a year's time.

(2) Endometrial thickness between 6 and 9 mm is classified as suspicious; control examination is recommended in 3–6 months' time.

(3) Endometrial thickness of 10 mm and more is classified as pathological; we recommend that the patient undergoes histological clearing through dilatation and curettage.

Sonographic assessment of endometria in postmenopausal women with hormonal replacement therapy is a completely different matter. In these women, it can be assumed that, as in the premenopause, endometrial thickness can reach 20 mm. Therefore, we recommend the following clinical procedure, which has proved successful in our routine:

(1) Endometrial thickness up to 10 mm is regarded as a normal finding; no further measurements are recommended; all patients with hormonal replacement therapy are advised to undergo sonographic checks of the endometrium in 6 months' time.

(2) Endometrial thickness between 10 and 20 mm is classified as suspicious. After administration of an oral gestagen, subsequent to the withdrawal bleeding, a second sonographic examination is carried out. If the endometrium still measures more than 10 mm, dilatation and curettage is recommended. With endometrial thickness of less than 10 mm, control examinations in 6 months' time are recommended.

(3) With endometrial thickness of 20 mm or more, primary dilatation and curettage is recommended on grounds of the unusual thickness. This procedure does not apply, however, to asymptomatic patients with hormonal replacement therapy, but only to patients with bleeding as well.

Generally, the endometrium of all postmenopausal women should be assessed vaginosonographically before the onset of hormonal replacement therapy. We differentiate between endometrial slow responders and fast responders[32]. Therefore, it seems to be important to perform a second vaginosonographic examination of the endometrium 3–6 months after commencement of the replacement therapy.

Endometrial findings under hormonal replacement therapy

The decrease of estrogen production in the postmenopause appears histologically as atrophy of the endometrium. The endometrium of postmenopausal women contains only very thin epithelial cells with blunt microvilli. The blood vessels have an extremely thin and delicate wall. Ruptures of the blood vessels or of the surface of the epithelia indicate that bleeding has occurred; due to the small amount of blood loss, however, this bleeding is clinically asymptomatic[33]. Glands are seldom found; they are either cystic and dilated or atrophic and show little secretion or no secretion at all[34]. The stroma cells are either small and scarcely developed or they are totally absent.

Although the endometrium is in a state of rest and the mitosis ratio is low, even in the menopause the uterus still has progesterone and estrogen receptors, which have the same characteristics as in the premenopause[35,36]. This is the reason that, even in the atrophic endometrium, a considerable and immediate stimulation of DNA synthesis in the epithelium is produced by replacement therapy with estrogens[37]. The elevated mitosis ratio in the glands, in the stroma and in the blood vessels leads to rapid growth of the endometrium. This occurs faster, according to the level of estrogen dosage and the duration of treatment. Thus, a normal and mature proliferative endometrium with both types of epithelial cells (secretory and cilial) can be found after 15–20 days of treatment with 1.25 mg conjugated estrogens. The microscopic picture presents pseudo-stratified, tubular glands, surrounded by many stroma cells[33].

The endometrium does not present a homogeneous picture; in proliferated areas, high enzyme activities can be observed, which may lead to increased focal proliferation. It is beyond doubt that there is a causal relationship between the long-term (i.e. uninterrupted by gestagen therapy) estrogen effect and the occurrence of a glandular–cystic hyperplasia. This may develop, under certain circumstances, into an adenomatous, then to an atypical hyperplasia and finally to a potentially malignant degeneration.

Development of a hyperplasia can be prevented and a pre-existing glandular–cystic or adenomatous hyperplasia can be eliminated by regular administration of gestagens[38]. For this purpose, it is important that the receptor mechanisms in the endometrium are intact. The quantity of progesterone receptors decreases with regard to increasing atypia. The success rate of gestagen therapy for hyperplasia amounts to 70%; it corresponds with the proportion of positive progesterone receptors in tissue specimens[39]. Under the effect of gestagen, the glandular epithelium is transformed into cylindrical, secretory glands, which are separated by larger stroma cells.

Whereas in untreated postmenopausal women the incidence of endometrial carcinoma is 2–3 per 1000[40], the incidence of endometrial carcinoma under estrogen therapy is significantly elevated, amounting to 3.6 per 1000[40–42]. There is no difference between cyclic and continuous estrogen therapy[38,41]. If the duration of therapy with conjugated estrogens is regarded as a risk factor, therapy of less than 1 year does not imply an elevated risk in comparison with non-treated women. However, after 1–4 years of therapy, there is an elevated risk of 2.9, after 5–9 years of 5.9 and after more than 10 years of 10 times the normal risk[42]. This can be minimized by giving gestagen for 10–13 days per cycle[43]. With gestagen therapy, the risk is even considerably below that of non-treated postmenopausal women.

Sonographic findings

Vaginosonography as a screening method enables us to survey the postmenopausal endometrium. Whilst the sonographic appearance of the cyclic endometrial changes in the premenopause has been widely examined, there are few clinical trials of sonographic changes of the endometrium under hormonal replacement therapy in the postmenopause[32,44,45]. According to Osmers and colleagues[46], the normal thickness of the endometrium in the postmenopause without hormonal replacement therapy reaches a maximum of 0.8 cm. Treatment with estrogens and gestagens leads to proliferation and secretory transformation of the endometrium even in the early postmenopause; as in the premenopause, this can be visualized sonographically.

For this purpose, the examiner of a postmenopausal woman should have knowledge of the type of hormonal replacement therapy and of the day of the menstrual cycle, in order to be able to distinguish pathological endometrial findings. It seems that the best time of examination is in the early postmenstrual period. In women under estrogen replacement therapy or combined continuous estrogen–gestagen replacement therapy, thickness of the endometrium between 0.8 and 1.5 cm is suspicious; in these cases dosage of the hormonal therapy should be changed and it is recommended that a biopsy should be taken. Thickness of the endometrium surpassing 1.5 cm requires histological examination in any case[44].

Endometrial findings under tamoxifen therapy

Tamoxifen is an adjuvant therapy for patients with breast cancer in the postmenopause. A certain number of studies have shown, however, that the occurrence of endometrial polyps, endometrial carcinoma and endometrial hyperplasia is increased under tamoxifen therapy[47–50]. A randomized clinical trial has shown evidence of an

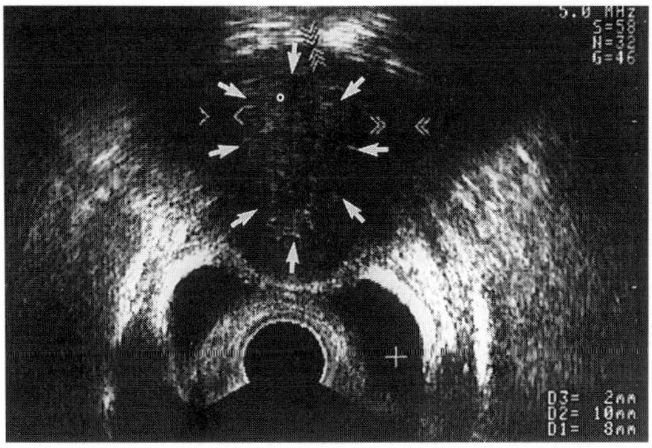

Figure 14 Irregularly cystic echogenic mass (arrows) in the uterine cavity under tamoxifen therapy. Histology: polyp without atypia

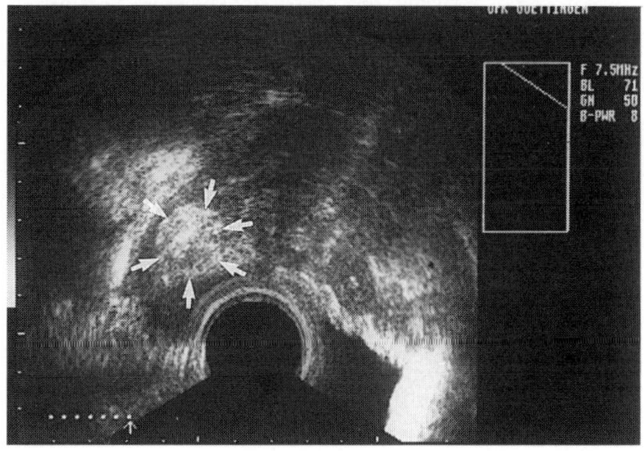

Figure 15 Pedunculated endometrial polyp in statu nascendi, which appears as a hypoechogenic mass in the cervical canal (white arrows). Histology: endometrial polyp without atypia

increased prevalence of endometrial carcinoma under tamoxifen therapy[51]. The sonographic appearance is multiform, however (Figure 14). In pathologically thickened endometrium, both homogeneously echogenic and echogenic tissues with small cysts can be observed[52]. Anteby and associates[53] report false-positive sonographic findings. When there were sonographic findings suspicious of a cystic and thickened endometrium, they turned out to be an atrophic endometrium under hysteroscopy and histology. The authors suggested that there might be a direct effect of the drug on the myometrium, which then undergoes cystic degeneration.

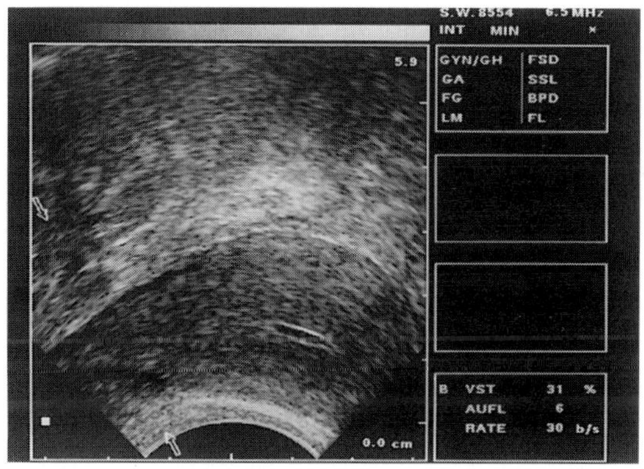

Figure 16 Small sero- or mucometra are frequently observed in postmenopausal uteri (16%). Without pathological changes of the endometrial layers, it is no sign of risk for endometrial carcinoma. Histology: atrophic endometrium

SONOGRAPHIC FEATURES OF BENIGN ENDOMETRIAL TUMORS

Even if, as mentioned above, there are no typical sonomorphological criteria for the assessment of benign or malignant intracavitary neoplasias, cystic endometrial polyps and glandular cystic hyperplasia present sonographically the most conspicuous and characteristic structures. In both conditions, small intracavitary cysts measuring between 1 and 3 mm, surrounded by echogenic tissue, can frequently be found. The variety of histomorphological results is underlined by a study by Schlief[54]; in classical endometrium with thin inclusion cysts the following findings can be expected: benign endometrial polyps, cystic hyperplasia, cystic atrophy or just atrophic endometrium. On the other hand, the endometrium with hypoechogenic areas, described as inhomogeneous, was characterized by the histological picture of endometrial carcinoma, atypic hyperplasia and atrophic endometrium (Figure 15).

Usually, fluid pools in the uterine cavity in the postmenopause are quite frequent. In our own population, we found fluid pools in the uterine cavity in 16% of all postmenopausal asymptomatic women (Figure 16). In narrow endometria there was no association, however, with pathological changes of the endometrium. It follows from this that serometra or mucometra alone cannot be considered as a risk factor for endometrial carci-

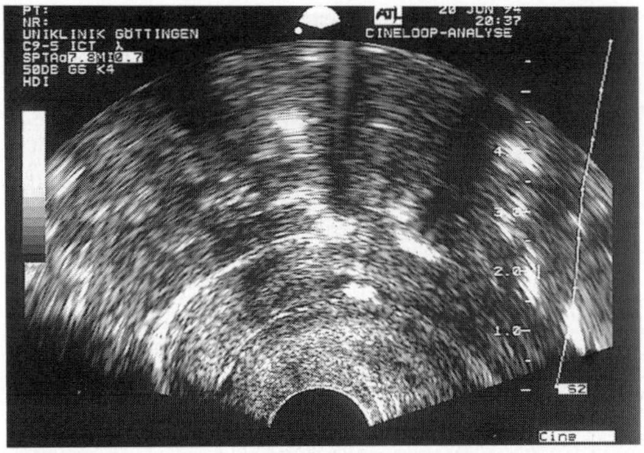

Figure 17 Hypoechogenic tumor of the internal os of the cervical canal due to a fibrous scar after several insertions of an intrauterine device

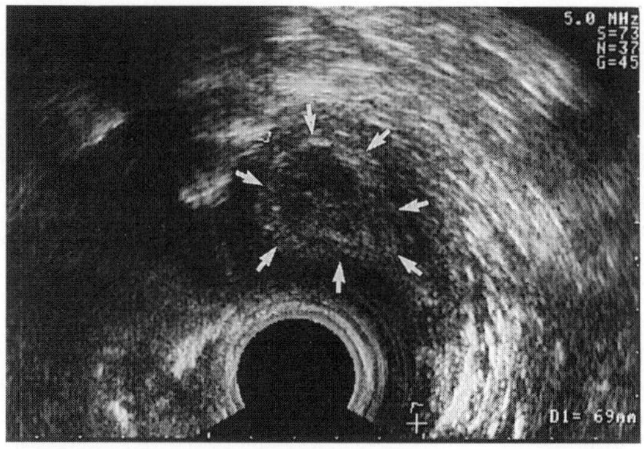

Figure 18 Complex hypoechogenic and hyperechoegenic mass in the uterine cavity of a retroflexed uterus (arrows). Histology: poorly differentiated adenocarcinoma of the uterus, stage Ic (FIGO)

noma; nor does this suggest the need for any clinical consequences such as dilatation and curettage. Indication for dilatation and curettage is given only when there are pathological endometrial findings at the same time.

In rare cases of osseous metaplasia of the endometrium, in ultrasound assessment an echogenic endometrium with distinct echo extinction phenomena was described[55]. Fibrosis and cicatrization of the endometrium present themselves as homogeneous, echogenic plaques with an echo extinction phenomenon. Being a frequent consequence of dilatation and curettage, renewed dilatation and curettage and the insertion of an intrauterine device, these changes can mainly be found at the height of the cervix/corpus boundary (Figure 17).

SONOGRAPHIC EVALUATION OF ENDOMETRIAL CANCERS

The ongoing endometrial carcinoma presents different features:

(1) The uterus is generally enlarged[6];

(2) The uterine cavity contains mainly echogenic or mixed hypoechogenic–hyperechogenic tumor[8,56,57] (Figure 18);

(3) The tumor most often grows asymmetrically into the myometrium[8] (Figure 19);

(4) Poorly-differentiated tumors may present a myometrial infiltration with hypoechogenic structures[58].

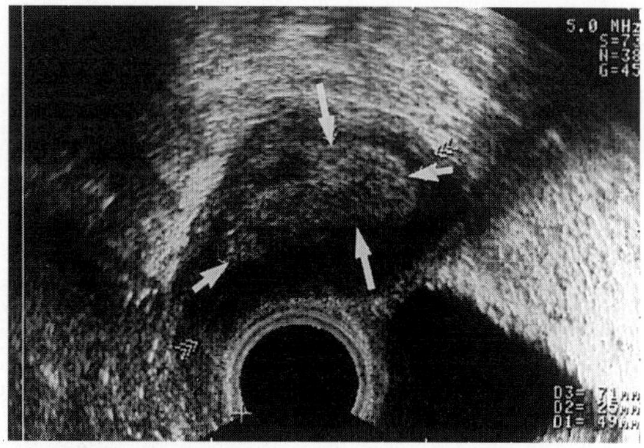

Figure 19 Asymmetrically growing echogenic tumor in the uterine cavity (arrows). Histology: endometrial cancer stage Ib (FIGO)

The myometrial infiltration itself is one of the most important prognostic risk factors when assessing endometrial carcinoma[57]. Many authors have tried to determine the depth of myometrial infiltration and of cervical invasion by means of transabdominal sonography[58–62]. The transabdominosonographically determined myometrial depths of infiltration have been confirmed histologically in 70%[58] to 80%[59] of cases. The transabdominosonographic assessment of cervical infiltration, however, has been difficult, and Thorvinger and colleagues[62] reported a sensitivity of only 25%.

Transvaginal sonography is vastly superior to the transabdominal route in these cases. Up to 80% of all infiltrating tumors are more echogenic than the myometrium[58], whilst the rest are less

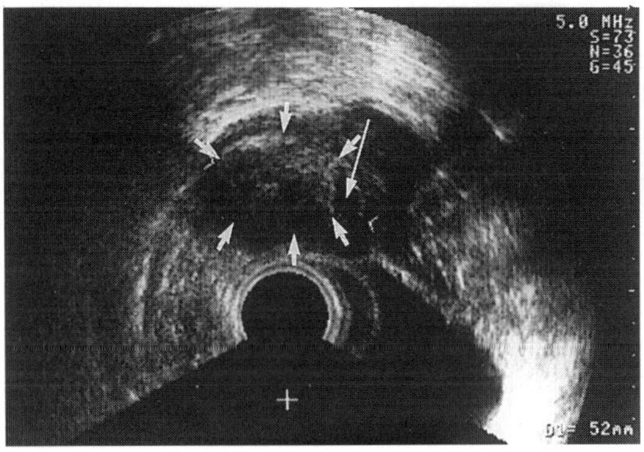

Figure 20 The mainly echogenic tumor of the endometrium is in contrast to the adjacent hypoechogenic myometrium. The asymmetrical growth of the histologically clarified endometrial cancer (short white arrows) is underlined by the presence of the small serometra (long white arrow)

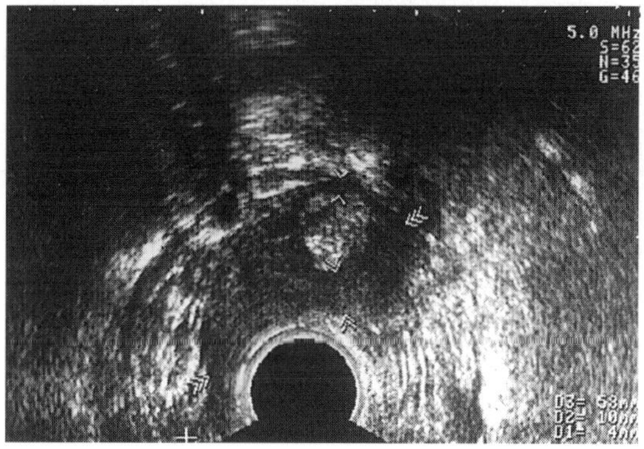

Figure 21 Echogenic endometrial tumor in the fundal part of the uterus. Histology: well-differentiated endometrial cancer stage Ic (FIGO)

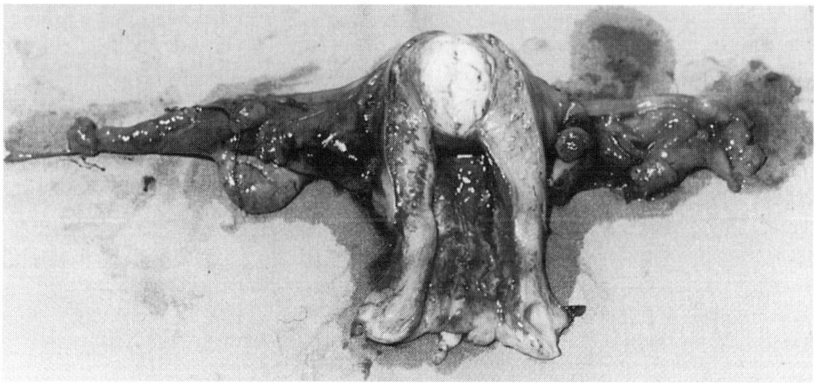

Figure 22 Same tumor as shown in Figure 21. Note the good correspondence between sonographic depiction and macroscopic appearance

echogenic than the surrounding tissue[56] (Figure 20). There seems to be a relation between the loss of echogenicity and a low tumor grading[56,58]. The myometrial infiltration, measured by transvaginal sonography, corresponds very well with the histologically verified infiltration of the myometrium[57,59,63] (Figures 21 and 22). In 75% of 76 vaginosonographically assessed endometrial carcinomas of stage Ia–IIb, we found a complete correspondence between sonography and the histological results. Of the tumors, 12% had been overestimated and 13% had been underestimated. However, we had not wrongly classified one single tumor of stage I as a tumor of stage II. Although at first sight an error rate of 25% seems to be high, the maximum discrepancy between sonographically and histologically measured tumor–serosa distance is about 4 mm. The overall tendency of overestimating the myometrial infiltration of the endometrial carcinoma is lower with vaginosonography than with transabdominal sonography[20,58,59]. It is worth mentioning that assessibility of myometrial infiltration is excellent with endoluminal hysterography[64,65]. As this is an invasive examination technique, however, it has not yet gained acceptance.

The sonographic prerequisites are less favorable when it comes to assessment of parametrial infiltration. For diagnosis of tumor recurrence, both vaginosonography and transrectal sonography are appropriate, especially in patients with vaginal stenosis or shortened vagina after operations or radiation[66,67]. Sonographically guided fine-needle biopsy may considerably facilitate finding the right diagnosis if tumor recurrence in the small pelvis is suspected. In contrast to the primary tumor, the tumor recurrence of the endometrial carcinoma appears as an echogenic, frequently well-vascularized space-occupying lesion.

References

1. Cornet, D., Giacomini, P., Pereira-Coelho, A. and Salat-Baroux, J. (1986). Etude échographique de l'epaisseur de l'endomiètre au cours des cycles spontanés et stimulés. *J. Gynecol. Obstet. Biol. Reprod.*, **324**, 621–5
2. Fleischer, A. C., Kalemaris, G. C. and Entman, S. S. (1986). Sonographic depiction of the endometrium during normal cycles. *Ultrasound Med. Biol.*, **12**, 272–81
3. Osmers, R., Völksen, M., Rath, W. and Kuhn, W. (1989). Die Vaginalsonographie: Eine Screeningmethode zur Früherkennung von Ovarialtumoren und Endometriumkarzinomen. *Arch. Gynecol. Obstet.*, **245**, 602–6
4. Randall, J. M., Fisk, N. M., McTavish, A. and Templeton, A. A. (1989). Transvaginal ultrasound assessment of endometrial growth in spontaneous and hyperstimulated menstrual cycles. *Br. J. Obstet. Gynaecol.*, **96**, 954–9
5. Schurz, B., Eppel. W., Huber, J. C. and Reinold, E. (1989). Vaginosonographische Darstellung des Endometriums postklimakte rischer Frauen. *Ultraschall*, **9**, 37–40
6. Osmers, R., Völksen, M., Rath, W. and Kuhn, W. (1990). Vaginosonographic detection of endometrial cancer in postmenopausal women. *Int. J. Gynecol. Obstet.*, **32**, 35–7
7. Fleischer, A. C., Kalemaris, G. C., Machin, J. E., Entman, S. S. and James, A. E. Jr (1986). Sonographic depiction of normal and abnormal endometrium with histopathologic correlation. *J. Ultrasound Med.*, **5**, 445–52
8. Sautter, T. (1990). *Transvaginalsonographie: Lehrbuch und Lehratlas*, pp. 45–60. (Stuttgart: Hippokrates)
9. Dallenbach-Hellweg, G. (1987). Histopathology of the Endometrium, 4th edn, pp. 86–92. (Berlin: Springer)
10. Ferenczy, A. (1987). Anatomy and histology of the uterine corpus. In Kurman, R. J. (ed.) *Blaustein's Pathology of the Female Genital Tract*, 3rd. edn, pp. 257–91. (New York: Springer)
11. Kurman, R. J. and Norris, H. J. (1987). Endometrial carcinoma. In Kurman, R. J. (ed.) *Blaustein's Pathology of the Female Genital Tract*, 3rd. edn, pp. 338–72. (New York: Springer)
12. Nasri, M.N., Shepherd, J. H., Setchell, M. E., Lowe, D. G. and Chard, T. (1991). Transvaginal ultrasound. A reliable basis for clinical management? Case reports. *Br. J. Obstet. Gynaecol.*, **98**, 485–6
13. Ghirardini, G., Montanari, M. and Gualerzi, C. (1990). Carcinoma and endometrial thickness (letter comment). *Lancet*, **335**, 1569–71
14. Varner, R. E., Sparks, J. M., Cameron, C. D., Roberts, L. L. and Soong, S. J. (1991). Transvaginal sonography of the endometrium in postmenopausal women. *Obstet. Gynecol.*, **78**, 195–9
15. Weigel, M., Schmitt, W. and Melchert, W. (1992). Die Eignung metrisch-struktureller Kriterien zur vaginosonographischen Beurteilung des postmenopausalen Endometriums. *Zent.bl. Gynkol.*, **114**, 420–4
16. Abu Hmeidan, F., Baier, D. and Bilek, K. (1991). Sonographic studies of patients with postmenopausal hemorrhage (endometrium/myometrium index). *Zent.bl. Gynkol.*, **113**, 707–12
17. Granberg, S., Wikland, M., Karlsson, B., Norström, A. and Friberg, L. G. (1991). Endometrial thickness as measured by endovaginal ultrasonography for identifying endometrial abnormality. *Am. J. Obstet. Gynecol.*, **164**, 47–52
18. Dorum, A., Kristensen, G. B., Langebrekke, A., Sornes, T. and Skaar, O. (1993). Evaluation of endometrial thickness measured by endovaginal ultrasound in women with postmenopausal bleeding. *Acta Obstet. Gynecol. Scand.*, **72**, 116–19
19. Karlsson, B., Granberg, S., Wikland, M., Ryd, W. and Norström, A. (1993). Endovaginal scanning of the endometrium compared to cytology and histology in women with postmenopausal bleeding. *Gynecol. Oncol.*, **50**, 173–8
20. Osmers R. G. W. and Kuhn, W. (1994). Endometrial cancer screening. *Curr. Opinion Obstet. Gynecol.*, **6**, 75–9
21. Coleman, B. G., Arger, P. H., Grumbach, K., Menard, M. K., Mintz, M. C., Allen, K. S., Arenson, R. L. and Lamon, K. A. (1988). Transvaginal and transabdominal sonography: prospective comparison. *Radiology*, **168**, 639–43

22. Osmers, R., Ulbrich, R., Rath, W., Völksen, M. and Kuhn, W. (1987). Vaginalsonographie, eine vielversprechende Methode zur Früherkennung von Endometriumveränderungen. Alete Wissenschaftlicher Dienst, *Berichte der Nordwestdeutschen Gesellschaft für Gynäkologie und Geburtshilfe*, 98 Tagung, pp. 323–6
23. Osmers, R., Völksen, M. and Schauer, A. (1990). Vaginalsonographie – Eine Methode zur Früherkennung des Endometriumkarzinoms? *Lancet* (German edition), **4**, 640–3
24. Smith, P., Bakos, O., Heimer, G. and Ulmsten, U. (1991). Transvaginal ultrasound for identifying endometrial abnormality. *Acta Obstet. Gynecol. Scand.*, **70**, 591–4
25. Creasman, W. T., Boronow, R. C., Morrow, C. P., Disaia, P. J. and Blessing, J. (1976). Adenocarcinoma of the endometrium: its metastatic lymphnode potential. *Gynecol. Oncol.*, **4**, 239–43
26. Creasman, W. T. and Weed, J. C. (1981). Carcinoma of endometrium (FIGO stages I & II): clinical features and management. In Copplesond, M. (ed.) *Gynecologic Oncology*, pp. 562–77. (Edinburgh: Churchill Livingstone)
27. Bachet, W., Brunner, P., Dodenhöfer, J. D. J. and Strobel, E. (1983). Diagnostische Treffsicherheit der Endometriumzytologie mit Prevical. *Geburtshilf. Frauenheilk.*, **43**, 11–14
28. Osmers, R., Völksen, M. and Kuhn, W. (1992). Evaluation of the endometrium in postmenopausal women by means of vaginal ultrasound. *Rev. Fr. Gynecol. Obstet.*, **87**, 309–15
29. Abu Hmeidan, F., Bilek, K., Baier, D., Nuwayhid, M. and Kade, R. (1992). Ultrasound assessment of the endometrium in early detection of endometrial cancer in high risk patients. *Zent.bl. Gynkol.*, **114**, 455–8
30. Seelbach-Göbel, B., Rempen, A. and Kristen, P. (1991). Vaginal sonography of the endometrium in postmenopause. Initial results of a prospective study. *Gynekol. Rundsch.*, **31** (Suppl. 2), 253–5
31. Maly, Z., Dorr, A. and Pilka, L. (1992). Results of transvaginal ultrasound screening for endometrial carcinoma in women at risk after menopause. *Cesk. Gynekol.*, **57**, 108–12
32. Meuwissen, J. H., van Langen, H., Moret, E. and Navarro-Morquecho, I. (1992). Monitoring of oestrogen replacement therapy by vaginosonography of the endometrium. *Maturitas*, **15**, 33–7
33. Flowers, C. E., Wilborn, W. H. and Hyde, B. M. (1983). Mechanisms of uterine bleeding in postmenopausal patients receiving estrogen alone or with a progestin. *Obstet. Gynecol.*, **61**, 135–43
34. Voet, R. L. (1983). End organ response to estrogen deprivation. In Buchsbaum, H.J. (ed.) *The Menopause*, pp. 9–22. (New York: Springer)
35. Tsibris, J. C. M., Cazenave, C. R., Cantor, B., Notelovitz, M., Kalra, P. S. and Spellacy, W. N. (1978). Distribution of cytoplasmic estrogen and progesterone receptors in human endometrium. *Am. J. Obstet. Gynecol.*, **132**, 449–54
36. Pellikka, P. A., Sullivan, W. P., Coulam, C. B. and Toft, D. O. (1983). Comparison of estrogen receptors in human premenopausal and postmenopausal uteri using isoelectric focusing. *Obstet. Gynecol.*, **62**, 430–4
37. Friedrich, E. R. and Meyer, J. S. (1982). Estrogen–progestin pharmacodynamics of the postmenopausal endometrium studied by thymidine labeling. *J. Obstet. Gynecol.*, **143**, 352–8
38. Astedt, B. (1982). On the role of estrogens in endometrial carcinogenesis. *Acta Obstet. Gynecol. Scand.*, (Suppl.), **106**, 33–5
39. Ehrlich, C. E., Young, P. C. M. and Cleary, R. E. (1981). Cytoplasmic progesterone and estradiol receptors in normal hyperplastic and carcinomatous endometria: therapeutic implications. *Am. J. Obstet. Gynecol.*, **141**, 539–46
40. Gambrell, R. D. (1980). Role of estrogens and progestogens in the etiology of breast and endometrial neoplasia. In Pasetto, N., Paoletti, R. and Ambrus, J. L. (eds.) *The Menopause and Postmenopause*, pp. 289–304. (Lancaster: MTP Press)
41. Hammond, C. B., Jelovsek, F. R., Lee, K. L., Creasman, W. T. and Parker, R. T. (1979). Effects of long-term estrogen replacement therapy. II. Neoplasia. *Am. J. Obstet. Gynecol.*, **133**, 537–47
42. Shapiro, S., Kelly, J. P., Rosenberg, L., Kaufman, D. W., Helmrich, S. P., Rosenshein, N. B., Lewis, J. L., Knapp, R. C., Stolley, P. D. and Schottenfeld, D. (1985). Risk of localized and widespread endometrial cancer in relation to recent and discontinued use of conjugated estrogens. *N. Engl. J. Med.*, **313**, 969–72
43. Studd, J. W. W., Thom, M. H., Paterson, M. E. L. and Wade-Evans, T. (1980). The prevention and treatment of endometrial pathology in postmenopausal women receiving exogenous estrogens. In Pasetto, N., Paoletti, R. and Ambrus, J. L. (eds.) *The Menopause and Postmenopause*, pp. 127–39. (Lancaster: MTP Press)
44. Lin, M. C., Gosink, B. B., Wolf, S. I., Feldesman, M. R., Stuenkel, C. A., Braly, P. S. and Pretorius, D. H. (1991). Endometrial thickness after menopause: effect of hormone replacement. *Radiology*, **180**, 427–32
45. Schurz, B., Metkam M., Heytmanek, G., Wimmer-Greinecker, G. and Reinold, E. (1988). Sonographic changes in the endometrium of climacteric women during hormonal treatment. *Maturitas*, **9**, 367–74
46. Osmers, R., Voelksen, M. and Schauer, A. (1990). Vaginosonography for early detection of endometrial cacinoma? *Lancet*, **335**, 1569–71
47. Malfetano, J. H. (1990). Tamoxifen-associated endometrial carcinoma in postmenopausal breast cancer patients. *Gynecol. Oncol.*, **39**, 82–4
48. Corley, C., Rowe, J., Curtis, M., Hogan, M.,

Novmoff, J. and Livolsi, V. (1992). Postmenopausal bleeding from unusual endometrial polyps in women on chronic tamoxifen therapy. *Obstet. Gynecol.*, **79**, 111–16

49. Neven, P., DeMuylder, X., VanBelle, Y., Venderick, G. and DeMuylder, E. (1990). Hysteroscopic follow-up during tamoxifen treatment. *Eur. J. Obstet. Gynecol. Reprod. Biol.*, **35**, 235–8
50. Cross, S. S. and Ismail, S. M. (1990). Endometrial hyperplasia in an oophorectomized woman receiving tamoxifen therapy (case report). *Br. J. Obstet. Gynaecol.*, **97**, 190–2
51. Fornander, T., Cedermark, B. and Mattson, A. (1989). Adjuvant tamoxifen in early breast cancer: occurrence of new primary cancers. *Lancet*, **1**, 117–20
52. Hulka, C. A. and Hall, D. A. (1993). Endometrial abnormalities associated with tamoxifen therapy for breast cancer: sonographic and pathologic correlation. *Am. J. Radiol.*, **160**, 809–12
53. Anteby, E., Yagel, S., Zacut, D., Palti, Z. and Hochner-Celnikier, D. (1992). False sonographic appearance of endometrial neoplasia in postmenopausal women treated with tamoxifen. *Lancet*, **340**, 433–4
54. Schlief, R. (1993). Diagnostic potential of intravenous contrast enhancement in various areas of cardiovascular Doppler ultrasound: Efficacy results of a multinational clinical trial with the galactose-based agent SH U 508 A. *Echocardiography*, **10**, 665–82
55. Acharya, U., Pinion, S. B., Parkin, D. E. and Hamilton, M. P. (1993). Osseous metaplasia of the endometrium treated by hysteroscopic resection. *Br. J. Obstet. Gynaecol.*, **100**, 391–2
56. Merz, E. (1988). *Sonographische Diagnostik in Gynäkologie und Geburtshilfe.* (Stuttgart: Thieme)
57. Schurz, B., Eppel, W., Egarter, C., Wenzl, R. and Reinold, E. (1989). Vaginosonographie in der Gynäkologie. *Ultraschall*, **10**, 90–7
58. Fleischer, A. C., Dudley, B. S., Entman, S. S., Baxter, J. W., Kalemeris, G. C. and James, A. E. Jr (1987). Myometrial invasion by endometrial carcinoma: sonographic assessment. *Radiology*, **162**, 307–10
59. Cacciatore, B., Lehtovirta, P., Wahlström, T., Ylänen, K. and Ylöstalo, P. (1989). Contribution of vaginal scanning to sonographic evaluation of endometrial cancer invasion. *Acta Oncol.*, **28**, 585–8
60. Gordon, A. N., Fleischer, A. C., Dudley, B. S., Drolshagan, L. F., Kalemeris, G. C., Partain, C. L., Jones, H. W. and Burnett, L. S. (1989). Preoperative assessment of myometrial invasion of endometrial adenocarcinoma by sonography (US) and magnetic resonance imaging (MRI). *Gynecol. Oncol.*, **34**, 175–9
61. Lehtovirta, P., Cacciatore, B., Wahlström, T. and Ylöstalo, P. (1987). Ultrasonic assessment of endometrial cancer invasion. *J. Clin. Ultrasound*, **15**, 519–24
62. Thorvinger, B., Gudmundsson, T., Horvath, G., Forsberg, L. and Holtas, S. (1989). Staging in local endometrial carcinoma. Assessment of magnetic resonance and ultrasound examinations. *Acta Radiol.*, **30**, 525–9
63. Bernaschek, G. (1987). Die endosonographische Diagnostik bei Uterusmalignomen. *Ultraschall*, **8**, 160–5
64. Becker, K. and Hötzinger, H. (1986). Die Hysterosonographie und ihre Bedeutung in der Diagnostik des Endometriumkarzinoms. *Geburtshilf. Frauenheilk.*, **46**, 693–6
65. Hötzinger, H. (1984). Durch Intrauterinsonographie optimierte intracavitäre Strahlentherapie bei Korpuskarzinomen. *Strahlentherapie*, **160**, 600–4
66. Bernaschek, G., Tatra, G. and Janisch, H. (1984) Die rektale Sonographie – eine Erweiterung dei Rezidivdiagnostik zervikaler Neoplasien. *Geburtshilf. Frauenheilk.*, **44**, 495–7
67. Giovannini, M., Rosello, R., Seitz, J.F., Houvenaeghel, G., Delpero, J. R. and Piana, L. (1989). L'échographie endorectale dans le bilan d'extension locorégionale des cancers gynécologique. *Presse Med.*, **18**, 128–9
68. Brandner, P., Gnirs, J., Neis, K. J., Hettenbach, A. and Schmidt, W. (1991). Der Stellenwert der Vaginosonographie in der non-invasiven Beurteilung des Endometruims am postmenopausalen Uterus. *Geburtshilfe Frauenheilkd.*, **51**, 734–40
69. Granberg, S. (1993). Personal communication
70. Schweighart, C., Schramm, T., Kurzl, R. and Stuckert-Klein, A. C. (1991). Endometruim-Karzinom: diagnostische Validitat eines vaginalsonographischen Screenings. *Gynakol. Rundsch.*, **31** (Suppl. 2), 256–8
71. Seelbach-Göbel, B. (1993). Personal communication

Fluid instillation into the uterine cavity 6

A. Suren, J. Puchta and R. Osmers

While in X-ray diagnosis the use of contrast media has been common, the use of contrast media in ultrasound diagnosis is of recent date. A hemato- or serometra produces a negative endogenous contrast in ultrasound, caused by the natural unfolding of the uterine cavity. This facilitates the delimitation and localization of intrauterine structures attached to the anterior or posterior wall. The sonographic visualization of the internal genital tract by means of exogenous media was used for the first time by Nannini and colleagues[1], Richman and colleagues[2] and Randolph and colleagues[3] in abdominosonographic examinations with intracervical fluid injection. With the uterine cavity filled with dextran or saline solution, it was easy to visualize such structures as submucous myoma or polyps, and to confirm the diagnosis afterwards by hysteroscopy.

Generally, all media having a different echogenicity from that of the human body can be used as contrast media. We differentiate between hypo- and hyperechogenic contrast media. Hypoechogenic contrast media (saline, Ringer or dextran solutions) may facilitate the detection of echogenic border surfaces. Instillation of normal saline solution into the uterine cavity may facilitate the localization of myoma or polyps, or the visualization of synechia. However, a fundamental disadvantage of hypoechogenic contrast media is that it is not possible to visualize phenomena of motion or flow. With hyperechogenic contrast media, i.e. media that enhance echo signals, it is possible to detect flow phenomena in the B-mode picture and to enhance Doppler signals. Therefore, these contrast media can be used both for the visualization of cavities and for function analysis. Since the pioneering work of Gramiak and Shah[4] and Meltzer and associates[5], it has been known that small bubbles of gas are very effective in reflecting ultrasonic waves. All commercial echo contrast media used at the present time are based on microbubbles[6].

Echo contrast media can be divided into three types, differing in their physical behavior:

(1) Fluids containing microbubbles (microfoam);

(2) Hollow microspheres filled with gas and made of special pretreated human albumin[7,8]; and

(3) Suspensions of microbubbles made of special galactose microparticles.

There are only few publications about the degradation of the hollow microspheres. They are probably eliminated by the reticuloendothelial system through phagocytosis. The acoustically active microstructures of the contrast media types I (microfoam) and III (suspension of microparticles) are degraded in the bloodstream.

Galactose microparticles are available as dry granules and have to be suspended in a watery transport solution by shaking before use. The commercial products Echovist® and Levovist® (Schering AG, Berlin) belong to this group of particles. The two substances work on the same principle. Galactose microparticle granules are suspended either in galactose solution (Echovist) or in sterile water (Levovist). After injection of this microbubble suspension containing galactose, cavities or blood become echogenic, until these microparticles have dissolved.

Echovist dissolves after intravenous injection, due to mixing with and dilution by the blood serum, before reaching the left heart. Therefore, it is suited to echocardiographic examination of the right heart by means of B-mode, sector scan and Doppler, as well as to examinations of the venous system. In addition, it is used as an indicator solution for sonographic visualization of the uterine cavity and of tube patency. After transcervical application and subsequent pertubation, temperature increase and dilution with body fluids lead to degradation and dissolution of the microparticles with following resorption of the galactose.

Levovist, compared with Echovist, is of higher intravascular stability, achieved by the addition of a physiological fatty acid. This leads to an increase of echogenicity in blood that will outlast – after intravenous injection – the passage of the lung and reach the arterial vascular bed. Thus, contrasting of the right and left heart cavities as well as of the whole arterial vascular bed can be achieved, provided the dosage is appropriate.

After dissolution of the acoustically active microparticles, the remaining galactose will be brought to its physiological, non-insulin-dependent degradation path, predominantly in the liver. Galactose is a non-toxic monosaccharide and is not allergenic. In the case of Levovist, the very small amount of physiological fatty acid does not lead to a measurable hyperlipemia. The small amount of microbubbles (about 100 μl) is excreted by breathing.

The acoustic characteristics of echo contrast media are important in connection with potential imaging artefacts, which might occur in the case of significant deviation from physiological values of sound velocity and dullness. Measured values of sound velocity of Echovist and Levovist in diagnostic concentrations are within the physiological range (1450 ± 50 m/s). Therefore, no relevant alteration of geometrical relations in the ultrasound picture is to be expected, not even when examining bigger spaces filled with contrast media. The sound attenuation caused by Levovist and Echovist depends on the concentration of the contrast media and the ultrasonic frequency. With diagnostic concentrations of 200 mg/ml for hysterosalpingocontrast sonography and 300 mg/ml for echocardiography, a rise of echogenicity without relevant shielding of subjacent structures in the image can be achieved. Principally, uncapsulated microbubbles have better dispersion than do corpuscular media. Shielding artefacts are not a fundamental problem, as they can be modified by dosage and mode of injection.

There is abundant experience from clinical studies in the areas of echocardiography, venous vascular systems and hysterosalpingocontrast sonography. Intravenous and local applications were well tolerated. In particular, there was no evidence of serious side-effects. There were no clinically relevant alterations of cardiovascular function nor of laboratory findings. Patients with galactosemia and patients in poor general condition had been excluded.

In general, tolerance of Echovist was good in clinical studies and it showed no substance-dependency risks. As in X-ray hysterosalpingography, patients without anesthesia may experience some pain. Immediately after the examination, there were more pain sensations from patients with impatent tubes than from patients with patent tubes. As in every pertubation, the risk of an ascending genital infection should be minimized by prior diagnostics and subsequent examination.

Absolute contraindications for instillation of fluids into the uterine cavity are acute inflammatory diseases of the genital system and, when using Echovist, galactosemia. Galactosemia is a metabolic disease with autosomal recessive inheritance. Due to a deficiency of galactose-1-phosphate uridyltransferase, galactose cannot be metabolized into glucose. Early onset and clinical symptoms of galactosemia are so drastic that it is almost impossible to be ignorant of the disease.

Instillation into the uterine cavity should be carried out postmenstrually until only day 10 of the cycle. For forensic reasons, a pregnancy test is recommended. A general or local infection should be excluded to the greatest possible extent by clinical findings, inspection, negative inflammatory symptoms and a degree of purity of 1 or 2.

After disinfection of the vagina, a small balloon catheter (Charr 6–8) is inserted into the cervical canal up to the internal os. The catheter is blocked with about 1 ml of saline solution. According to the investigator's experience, other sets and catheters may also be suitable: Schultze's or Cohen's set, Zinnert-catheters, Bard-catheters or Ackrad-catheters.

Under vaginosonographic control, the uterine cavity is filled with liquid, followed by intermittent injections up to a total volume of 10–20 ml. At the moment of injection, the uterine cavity is distended to a maximum degree and can be well delimited for assessing intrauterine structures as well as structures attached to the uterine wall. At the moment of injection, some patients experience discomfort, especially when there is tubal obstruction, so that complaints may indicate tubal pathology.

For exact differentiation of uterine structures the womb has to be scanned in longitudinal sections from median to lateral and vice versa. The balloon catheter or the cone of the application set is localized before following the normally smooth contour of the endometrium posteriorly and anteriorly until reaching the fundus. Special attention has to be paid to structures protruding into the uterine cavity. When rotating, special attention is given to possible increase or decrease of the endometrial thickness and to a possible up or down movement of the upper boundary of the uterine cavity which may give some evidence of malformation. Finally, the Douglas pouch is checked for retrouterine free fluid, which may give proof of tubal patency, at least on one side. Examination is continued of transverse sections of the uterus. The sonographic cross-sections are laid from the cervix to the fundus and vice versa, while continuing the fluid injections. In the domain of the fundus, special attention is paid to uterine malformation and similar phenomena.

By using Echovist in combination with transvaginal examination techniques, we now have an alternative for X-ray hysterosalpingography[9,10]. Besides the diagnosis of uterine malformations, transvaginal application and pertubation of Echovist allow us to detect tubal patency. Contrary to conventional methods such as hysterosalpingography or chromolaparoscopy/hysteroscopy, the advantage of this method lies in the absence of any radiation exposure, allergic reactions to contrast media or operative risks.

The sonographically normal uterine cavity

The contour of the cavity, filled with hypo- or hyperechogenic contrast media, is normally spindle- or club-shaped and smooth. This is true for anteflexion and retroflexion of the uterus (Figures 1 and 2). When the probe is rotated in the longitudinal section from the right to the left tubal exits, the boundary of the fundus should be seen at the same height on either side. If not, this could indicate a uterine malformation. In the frontal section, the upper segment of the uterine cavity has the shape of an ellipse or a dumb-bell, narrowing towards the cervix.

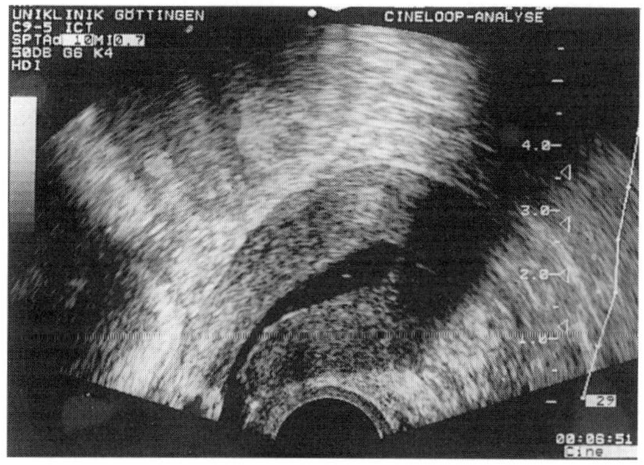

Figure 1 Normal uterus with normal endometrium in longitudinal section, filled with hypoechogenic contrast medium (saline solution)

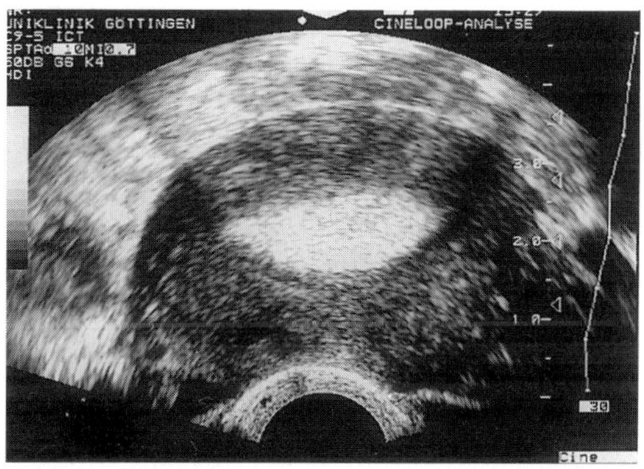

Figure 2 Normal uterus with normal cavity in transverse section, filled with hyperechogenic contrast medium (Echovist®)

The sonographically abnormal uterine cavity

Sometimes during injection, thin floating structures coming from the endometrium and projecting into the lumen can be seen. These are detached strips of mucosa, which are of no pathological significance (Figure 3).

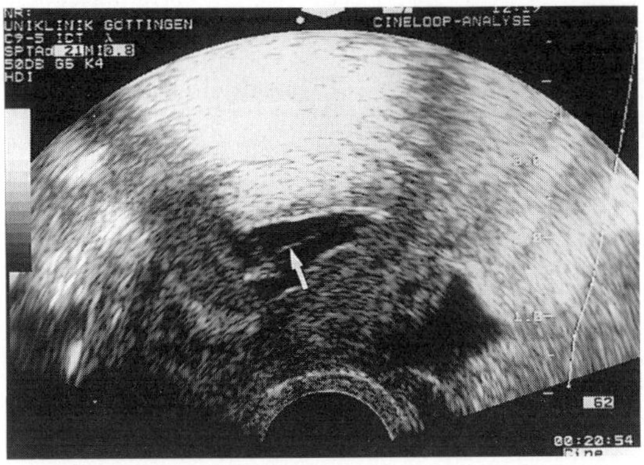

Figure 3 Corpus uteri with septa (arrow) in longitudinal section, after instillation of contrast medium

Immobile structures are suspicious. Rigid, thin connections between the uterine anterior and posterior walls can be synechiae. Round, hyporeflective, sessile structures are uterine polyps (Figures 4, 5 and 6) or submucous myoma (Figure 7). The predictive value of contrast sonography in detection of uterine pathology in comparison with hysteroscopy has been confirmed[3]

Localization and differentiation of intramural and submucous myoma, including their distance from the uterine cavity, can be much better assessed with instillation of contrast media than with other techniques[11] (Figures 8 and 9). It is possible to assess preoperatively if there is

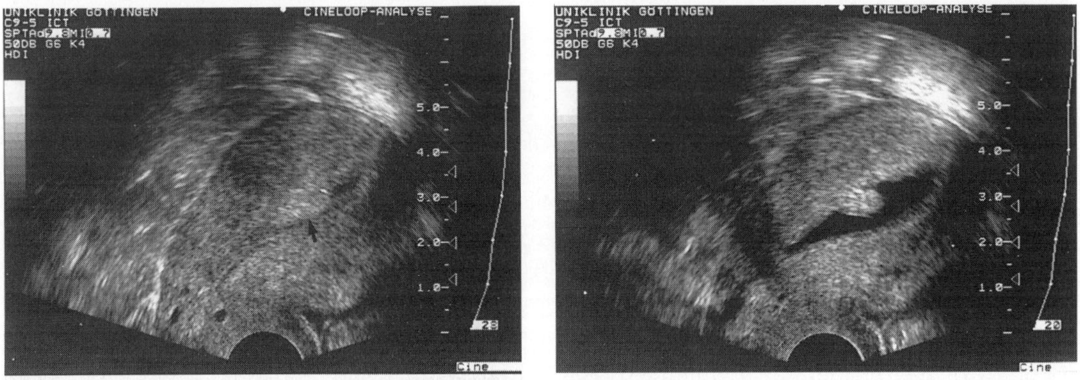

Figure 4 Corpus uteri with a polyp (arrow) in the uterine cavity in longitudinal section before (left) and after (right) instillation of normal saline solution. Before it cannot be determined whether the polyp is related to the posterior or anterior wall, but after it can be seen that the polyp is attached to the posterior wall

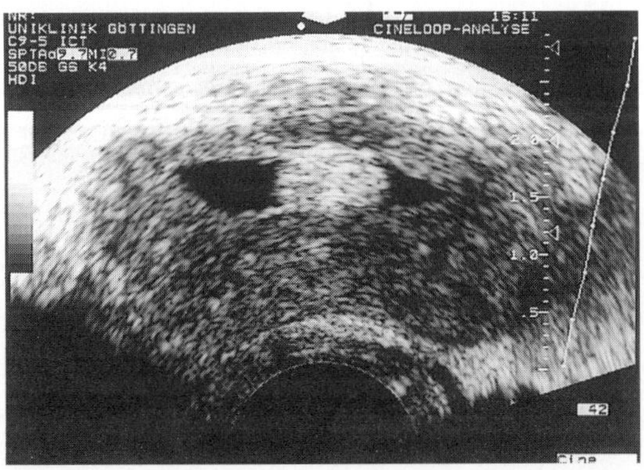

Figure 5 Uterus with polyp (transverse section)

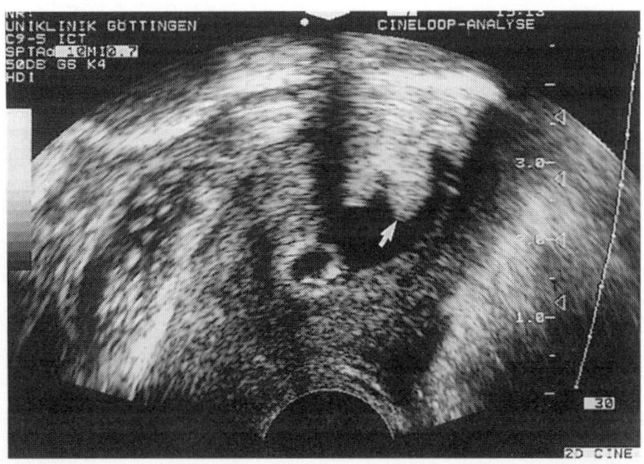

Figure 6 Uterus with polyp (arrow) in the area of the fundus in longitudinal section. Precervically, the balloon of the Foley catheter can be seen

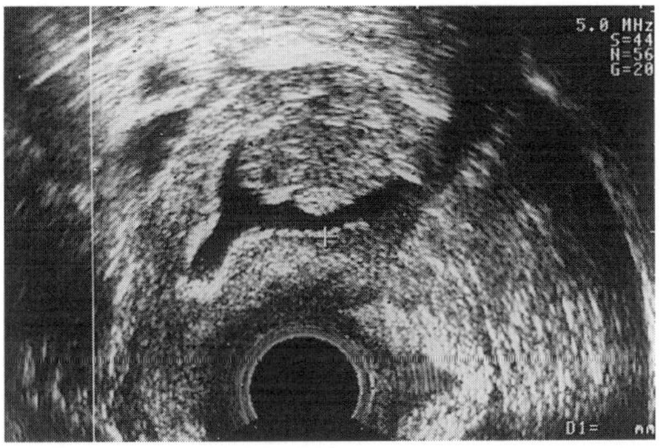

Figure 7 Uterus with submucous myoma in the area of the posterior wall of the fundus (longitudinal section)

sufficient distance between the capsule of the myoma and the uterine cavity and thus to estimate beforehand whether or not the uterine cavity needs to be opened. With submucous myoma, the depth of penetration of the nodules into the myometrium can be determined. This imaging of uterine wall layers facilitates the decision of which therapy to choose: drug therapy, endoscopy or hysteroscopy. The predictive value of abdominal ultrasound screening for the detection of malformations has been judged by different groups[12,13]. Serious malformations such as bicornuate uterus will be noticed immediately and diagnosed correctly[13]. However, mild defects such as arcuate uterus or bipartite uterus will be noticed rather seldom. In this respect, radiological hysterosalpingography was superior. With the possibility of spreading apart the uterine walls by means of liquid or contrast media injected into the cavity, however, we now have conditions similar to those in hysterosalpingography.

In the normal uterus, the cranial boundary of the fundus moves up only a little when the probe is rotated from the median longitudinal section towards the lateral; the thickness of the myometrium in the region of the fundus remains about the same. In the cross-section of the uterus, from caudal to cranial, normally there is a club-shaped structure in the uterine cavity and, finally, only the comma-shaped echoes of the lateral corner of the uterine cavity can be seen. In the arcuate uterus, the uterine fundus moves cranially when the probe is guided in the longitudinal section from median to lateral, and vice versa. In the cross-section, two spindle-shaped, hyporeflective structures appear, one lying beside the other like a 'cat-eye phenomenon'. In the longitudinal section of the bipartite uterus, there is no visible up or

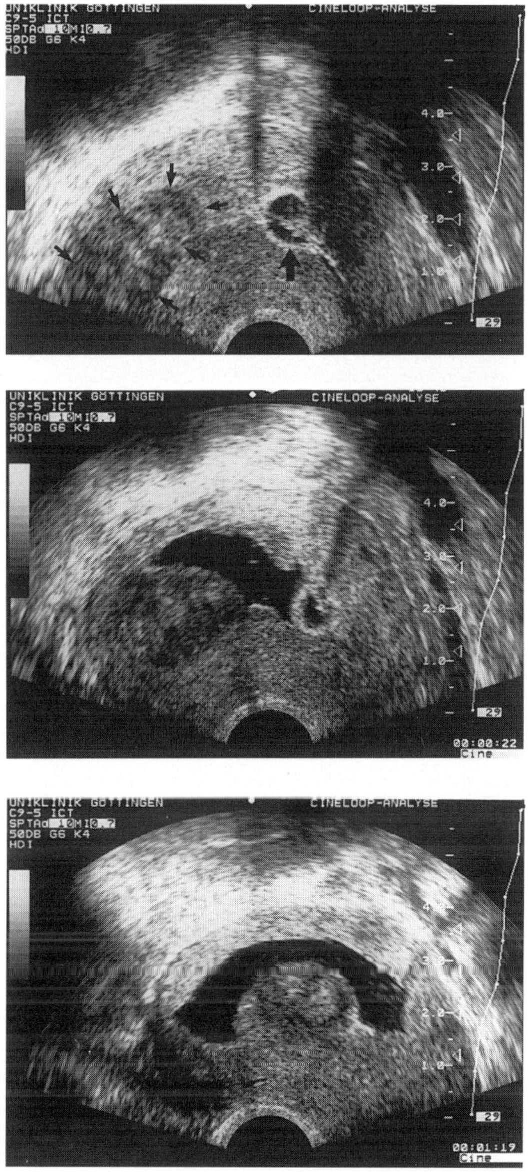

Figure 8 Retroflexed uterus with hypodense myoma (small arrows) and precervical balloon catheter (large arrow). Localization (submucous or intramural; posterior or anterior wall) cannot be determined without contrast medium (top). Beginning of instillation (middle) and complete filling of the uterine cavity (bottom). Submucous myoma in the posterior wall

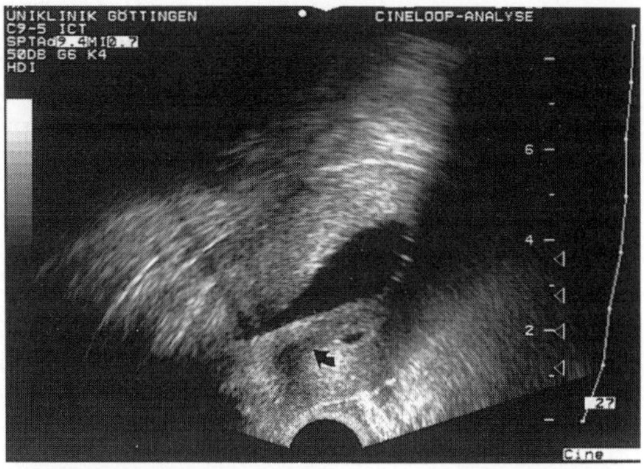

Figure 9 Corpus uteri with the peduncle (arrow) of the myoma in statu nascendi (longitudinal section)

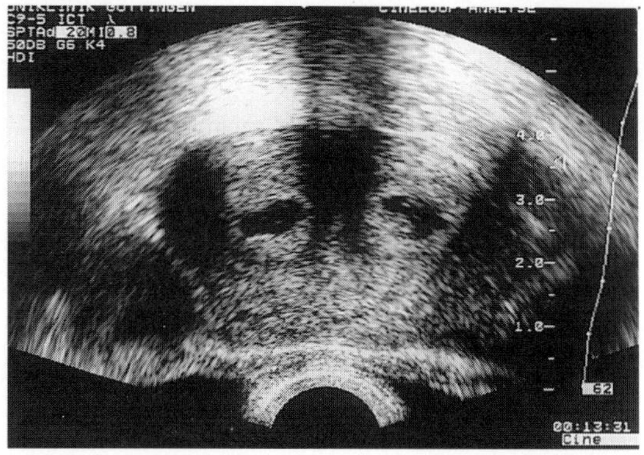

Figure 10 Bicornuate uterus (transverse section)

down movement of the outer boundary of the fundus when the probe is rotated laterally; but when it is rotated towards the median, an increase of the thickness of the uterine wall is evident. In the cross-section, a figure similar to the 'cat-eye phenomenon' can be observed, with the exception that the hyporeflective areas are oval and broader in the anterior–posterior direction.

In distinct malformations such as a bicornuate or double uterus, movement of the fundus during rotation is still more obvious. In the frontal section with the bicornuate uterus in extension, a Y-shaped formation can be seen. In the cross-section with the uterus in antiflexion, a star-shaped contrast figure of the cavity echo is apparent. In the cross-section of the uterus, the cavity echoes diverge widely. The apparent malformation of the bicornuate uterus can already be estimated by basic ultrasound from the median excavation and, more specifically during the luteal phase, from the endometrium echo as a guiding structure.

Bicornuate unicollis uterus with rudimentary horn on either side is a special case. If the connection between the two horns is missing, it is possible to fill the main horn only, or one cavity and one tube. The indication for a second cavity is given by the endometrial echo of the rudimentary horn[14].

References

1. Nannini, R., Chelo, E., Branconi, F., Tantini, C. and Scarselli. G. F. (1981). Dynamic echohysteroscopy: a new diagnostic technique in the study of female infertility. *Acta Eur. Fertil.*, **12**, 165–71
2. Richman, T. S., Viscomi, G. N., de Cherney, A., Polan, M. L. and Alcebo, L. O. (1984). Fallopian tubal patency assessed by ultrasound following fluid injection. *Radiology*, **152**, 507–10
3. Randolph, J. R., Ying, Y. K., Maier, D. B., Schmidt, C. I. and Riddick, D. H. (1986). Comparison of real-time ultrasonography, hysterosalpingography and laparoscopy/hysteroscopy in the evaluation of uterine abnormalities and tubal patency. *Fertil. Steril.*, **46**, 828–32
4. Gramiak, R. and Shah, P. M. (1968). Echocardiography of the aortic root. *Invest. Radiol.*, **3**, 356–66
5. Meltzer, R. S., Tickner, G., Sahines, T. P. and Popp, R. L. (1980). The source of ultrasound contrast effect. *J. Clin. Ultrasound*, **8**, 121
6. Ophir, J. and Parker, K. J. (1989). Contrast agents in diagnostic ultrasound. *Ultrasound Med. Biol.*, **15**, 319–33
7. Reisner, A. S., Shapiro, J. R., Amico, A. F. and Meltzer, R. S. (1989). Contrast agents for myocardial perfusion studies. In Meerbaum, S. and Meltzer, R. (eds.) *Myocardial Contrast Two-dimen-*

sional Echocardiography, pp. 45–56. (Dordrecht: Kluwer)

8. Schlief, R. and Deichert, U. (1991). Hysterosalpingo-contrast sonography: results of a clinical trial with a novel US contrast medium in 120 patients. *Radiology*, **178**, 213–15
9. Deichert, U., Schlief, R., van de Sandt, M. and Juhnke, I. (1989). Transvaginal hysterosalpingo-contrast sonography (Hy-Co-Sy) compared with conventional tubal diagnostics. *Hum. Reprod.*, **4**, 418–24
10. Hüneke, B., Lindner, C. and Braendle, W. (1989). Untersuchung der Tubenpassage mit der vaginalen gepulsten Kontrastmittel-Doppler-Sonographie. *Ultraschall Klin. Prax.*, **4**, 192–8
11. Deichert, U., van de Sandt, M., Lauth, G. and Daume, E. (1988). Die transvaginale Hysterokontrastsonographie (HKSG). Ein neues diagnostisches Verfahren zur Differenzierung intrauteriner und myometraler Befunde. *Geburtshilf. Frauenheilk.*, **48**, 835–44
12. Valdes, C., Malni, S. and Malinak, L. R. (1984). Ultrasound evaluation of female genitaltract anomalies: a review of 64 cases. *Am. J. Obstet. Gynecol.*, **149**, 285
13. Nicolini, U., Belotti, M., Bonazzi, B., Zamberletti, D. and Candiani, G. B. (1987). Can ultrasound be used to screen uterine malformations? *Fertil. Steril.*, **47**, 89–93
14. Deichert, U. and Schlief, R. (1993). Untersuchungen von Uterus und Tuben durch tranvaginale Hystersalpingo-Kontrastsonographie (HKSG). In Deichert, U., Duda, V. and Schlief, R. (eds.) *Funktionelle Sonographie in Gynäkologie und Reproduktionsmedizin*, pp. 199–236. (Berlin: Springer-Verlag)

Sonographic appearance of the myometrium

7

D. Kulenkampff, J. Puchta and R. Osmers

NORMAL FINDINGS

The smooth muscles of the myometrium, shaped like a concertina barrier, appear sonographically as a homogeneous structure with moderate-level echotexture. In the median cross-section the uterus can be seen as a pear-shaped organ, which can be divided into corpus, isthmus and cervix (Figure 1). The outer boundary of the uterus is the perimetrium, imaging in sonography as a hyperechogenic line. In the center of the uterus can be seen – depending on the day of the menstrual cycle – a more or less distinct hyperechogenic stripe of endometrium (Swiss cheese endometrium).

Measurement of the uterus in the sagittal plane can be carried out either by determination of the portio–fundus distance or – in special cases – by separate measurement of cervix and corpus uteri (Figure 2). This measurement is supplemented by determination of the largest anterior–posterior diameter of the corpus uteri, and of the largest transverse diameter of the corpus in the same tomolevel in which the ovaries are viewed (Figure 3).

The position of the uterus in the pelvic space (anteflexion, retroflexion or extension) can be judged, as well as sinistro- or dextroposition. These different positions are of no pathological value, but can be a sign of space-occupying lesions in the pelvis. The vaginal probe can be used tactually, and can, after careful movement of the uterus, give evidence of decreased motility, which may indicate possible intra-abdominal adhesions in the pelvic space. This can become more evident by moving the intestinal loops along the uterus with the vaginal probe.

Depending on parity and age, the uterus varies in aspect and size. Hata and colleagues[1] carried out measurements of volume in uteri of the newborn. They differentiated between volume of the corpus and the cervix, the latter measuring about three times the former. The cervix volume was found to be $3.65 \pm 1.36\,cm^3$, and the corpus volume $1.18 \pm 0.42\,cm^3$. The total volume of the uterus was $1.57\,cm^3$. Data for the infantile uterus from 1 year onward, reported by Deutinger and Bernaschek[2] were on average lower, due to the

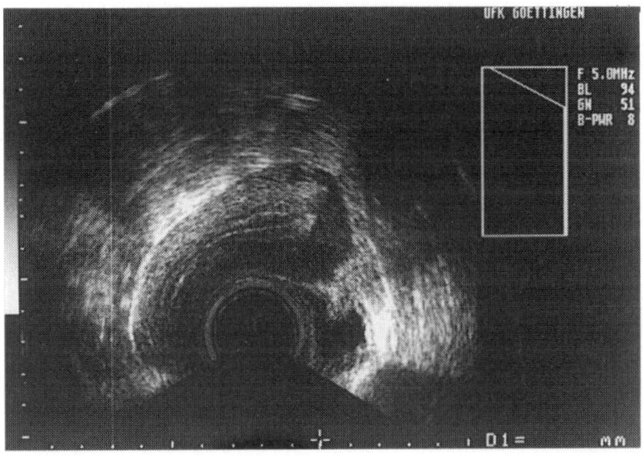

Figure 1 Anteflexed uterus with mid-cyclic endometrium and normal myometrium (longitudinal section)

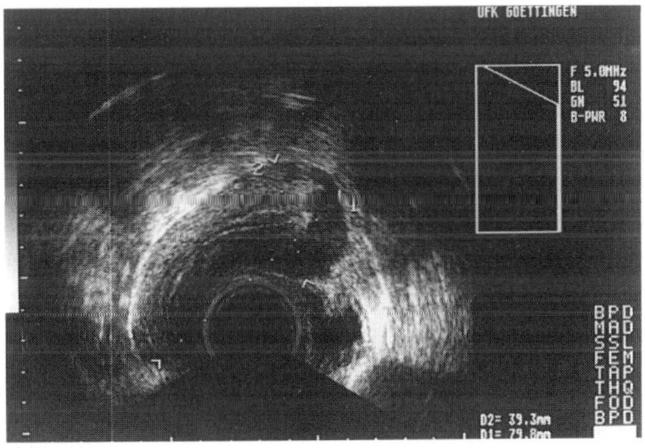

Figure 2 Measurement of the uterus: anterior–posterior diameter (D2) and longitudinal diameter (D1)

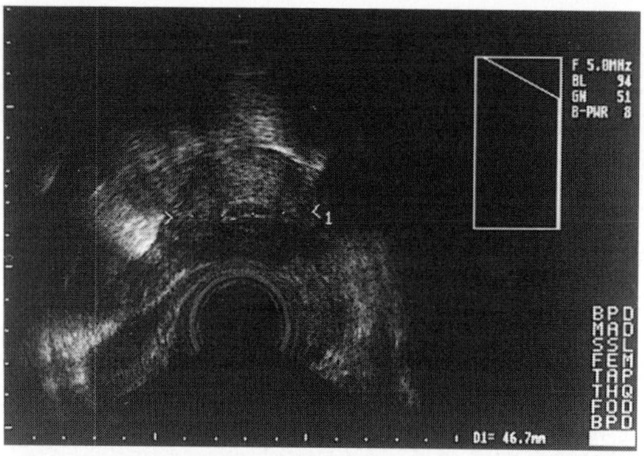

Figure 3 Measurement of the transverse diameter (D1) of the uterus

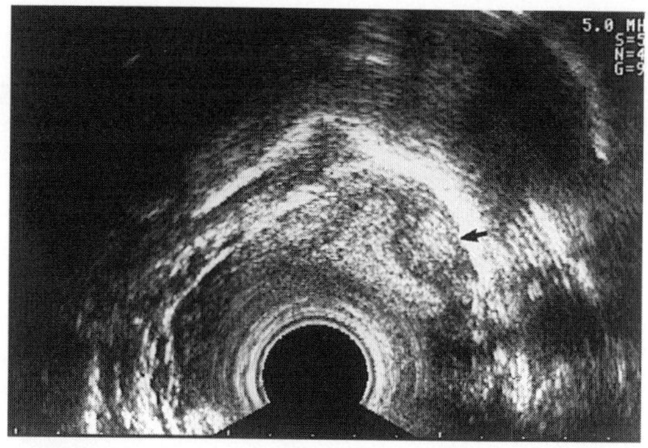

Figure 4 Arcuate uterus, with discrete fundal impression of the myometrium (arrow). Depiction of the endometrium in both cornua (longitudinal section inclined laterally)

decreasing estrogen effect. In these studies, the volume calculated by median length × anterior–posterior × breadth of the uterus was 2.4 × 0.8 × 1.0 cm³. The team of Orsini[3] showed that the size of the uterus remained stable until the age of 7 years, and that the size of the cervix predominated over the size of the corpus. From the age of 7 onward, there is continuous growth of the womb, the relation between the cervix and corpus equalizing. Gurr and associates[4] showed that there is a significant increase of growth around the time of the menarche. In menstruating nulliparae, the ratio of cervix to corpus has changed, with the corpus accounting for two-thirds of the uterine length.

According to Platt and co-workers[5], the average weight of the uterus in menstruating nulliparae is 60 ± 20 g. After at least one delivery, an average uterus weighs 121 ± 35 g. Within an ovulatory cycle, the uterus is subject to perceptible changes of size, with the smallest size around day 12 of the cycle and the maximum size shortly before menstruation[6].

After menopause, the size of the uterus/corpus decreases markedly, shrinking to average values of 4.5 × 1.5 × 2.5 cm³, with the cervix predominating over the corpus in the sense of elongation of the cervix.

SONOGRAPHIC FEATURES OF UTERINE MALFORMATIONS

The uterus arises from fusion of the Müllerian ducts. Different degrees of insufficient fusion of the Müllerian ducts lead to a great number of malformations, varying in type and extent[7]. The most common reduction deformity of the genital tract affects the uterus, but rather seldom the vagina or the ovaries. The overall incidence of fusion disorders of the Müllerian duct system is estimated at below 5%[8,9]. The majority of these malformations will not be recognized or diagnosed, as they are clinically asymptomatic. According to Rock[10], uterovaginal malformations can be divided into four categories:

- Type I Dysgenesis of the Müllerian ducts;
- Type II Vertical fusion disorders, such as transvaginal septa;
- Type III Lateral fusion disorders; and
- Type IV Complicated configurations of the Müllerian duct system, which cannot be classified.

The malformations summarized under type III account for the majority of malformations. By means of sophisticated sonographic diagnostics, a first diagnostic approach and classification is possible. Uterus didelphys, uterus unicornuatus, uterus bicornis (incomplete and complete), uterus arcuatus (Figure 4) and uterus septus (incomplete and complete) (Figure 5) can be summarized in this group.

In diagnosis of genital tract malformations, sonography as a non-invasive method is a con-

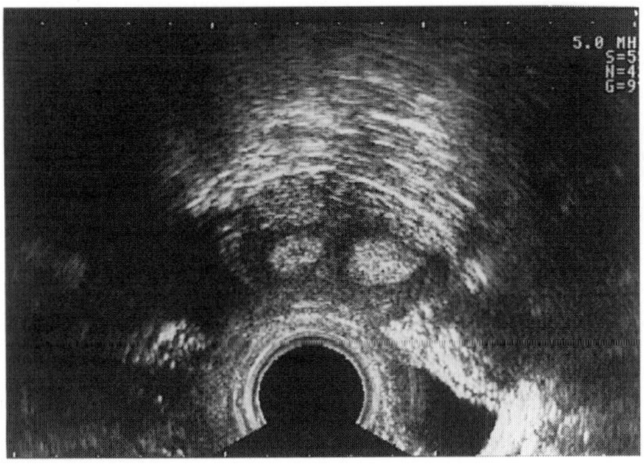

Figure 5 Septate uterus, with septum dividing the endometrium into two cavities (transverse section)

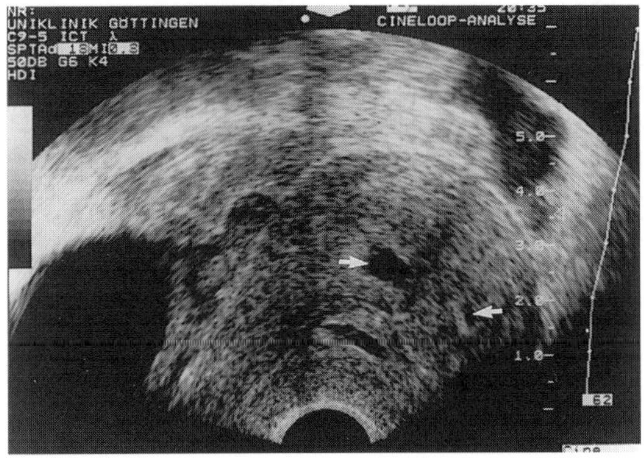

Figure 6 Transverse section showing uterine adenomyosis. Myometrium with hypodense areas (arrows) corresponding with cavities filled with blood

siderable step forward, and should in any case be applied before using other invasive methods such as hysterosalpingography, hysteroscopy or laparoscopy. Sonography can also be used in children and pregnant women. Transabdominal imaging of uterine anomalies is best carried out with the patient's bladder partly filled. This turns the uterus vertically to the abdominal wall and enables evaluation in the frontal longitudinal section. Best conditions are in the second half of the menstrual cycle with the endometrium being thick. From the endometrial structures in transverse, longitudinal, medial and paramedial sections, assignment of the different uterus anomalies is possible. Diagnosis can be difficult in the case of myoma or retroflexion of the uterus. As anomalies of the internal genitalia are associated in 20% of cases with anomalies of the urinary tract, thorough examination of the kidneys and the deferent urinary tract should be carried out.

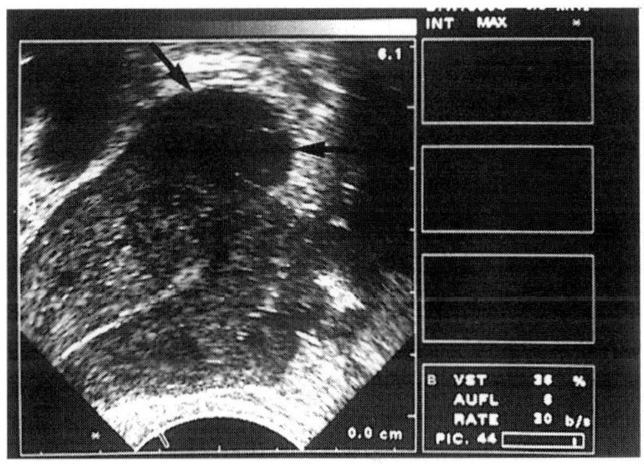

Figure 7 Longitudinal section showing uterine adenomyosis with protrusion of the posterior wall of the myometrium (arrows)

ADENOMYOSIS UTERI INTERNA

Adenomyosis uteri interna is characterized by growth of endometrial glands into the myometrium. The growth may be present throughout the uterus or only in a focal area, so that two different forms can be distinguished: diffuse and nodular adenomyosis. Depending on the literature consulted, the frequency of adenomyosis uteri interna differs between 5 and 70%[11].

Preoperative diagnosis of adenomyosis uteri interna is often difficult. An enlarged uterus, menorrhagia and/or dysmenorrhea can be clinical signs of adenomyosis uteri, provided there is no indication of leiomyomas or any other endometrial pathology. The diffuse form of adenomyosis uteri interna appears sonographically as a myohyperplastic uterus with a possible enhancement in the area of the posterior wall. In addition to the features mentioned above, the nodular form may present small, irregular cystic structures in the myometrium with a partially echogenic halo (Figures 6 and 7). Fedele and co-workers[12] could not find any changes that were related to the menstrual cycle; this would be due to the basal cell type of the uterine stroma and glandular tissue, which is not very hormone-sensitive[12]. Diagnosis of adenomyosis uteri interna can only be

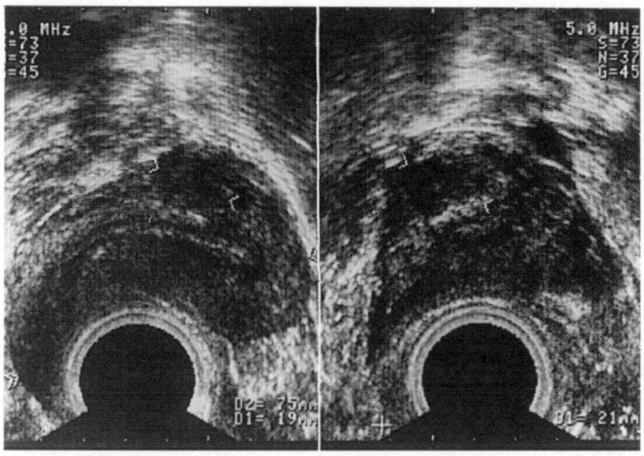

Figure 8 Anteflexed uterus with intramural myoma of the posterior wall, in longitudinal section (left) and transverse section (right)

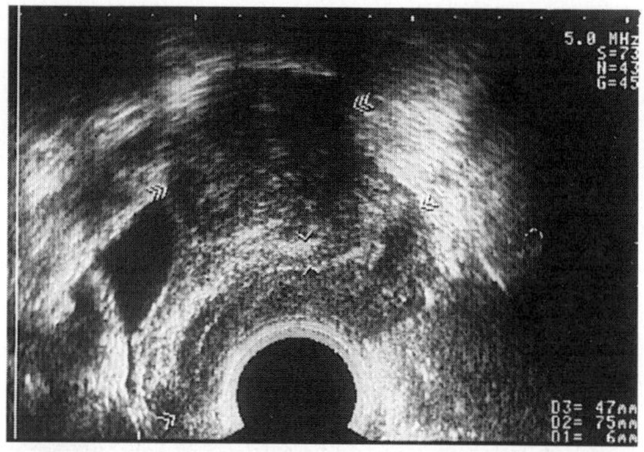

Figure 9 Subserous myoma of the posterior wall (longitudinal section)

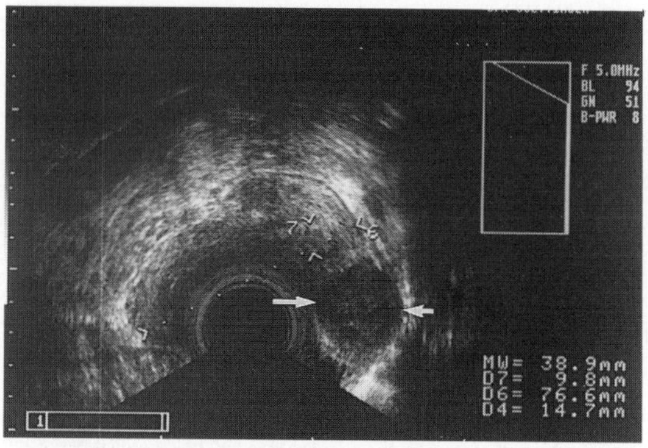

Figure 10 Subserous myoma (arrows) of the anterior wall (longitudinal section)

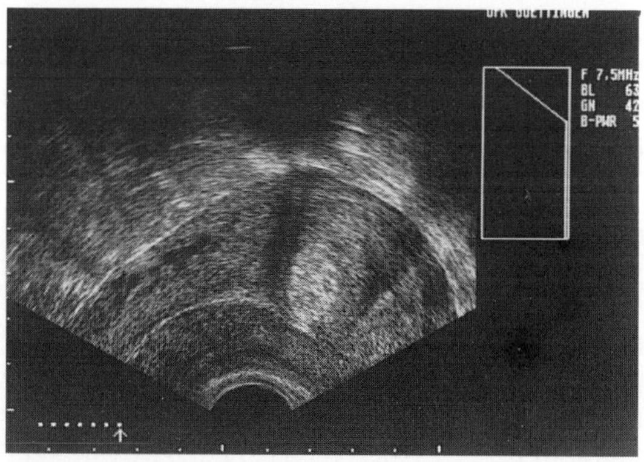

Figure 11 Submucous myoma of the posterior wall with lateral echo extinction (longitudinal section)

established on the grounds of clinical symptoms[13]. In these cases the sonomorphological picture can contribute to the diagnosis. In their study group, Fedele and associates[12] achieved a sensitivity of 80% and a specificity of 74% for the diagnosis of adenomyosis; the prevalence was 47%. These results were confirmed by Walsh and Bohlmann and their groups[14,15].

SONOGRAPHIC FEATURES OF LEIOMYOMAS

Myomas are tumors of smooth muscle with more or less connective tissue. Myomas are the commonest benign tumors of the uterus. Patients with myomas, who need treatment, contribute to about 10% of all gynecological patients[16]. In about 20% of all women over 30 years, myomas are multiple rather than solitary; 90% of myomas occur after the age of 30. Myomas before the age of 25 are very rare. Myomas grow in the generative phase of female life only. Growth of myomas has been shown to be estrogen-dependent. As myomas grow rather slowly, one has to be aware of malignancy in the case of rapid growth or growth in the postmenopause. The overwhelming majority of myomas are to be found in the corpus. In about 8%, they occur in the cervix[17]. Myomas can be localized intramurally (50%) (Figure 8), subserously (35%) (Figures 9 and 10), submucously (5%) (Figure 11) or in the pelvic ligaments (Figure 12).

In sonography, the uterus appears enlarged and irregularly outlined. Myomas present as round or oval space-occupying lesions. The typical capsule, developing from surrounding normal myometrium, can appear as a reflecting echo. The

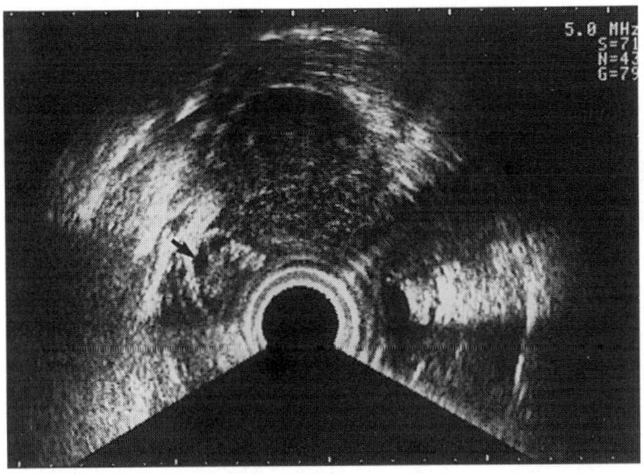

Figure 12 Intraligamentary myoma. The right ovary (arrow) is depicted laterally to the myoma

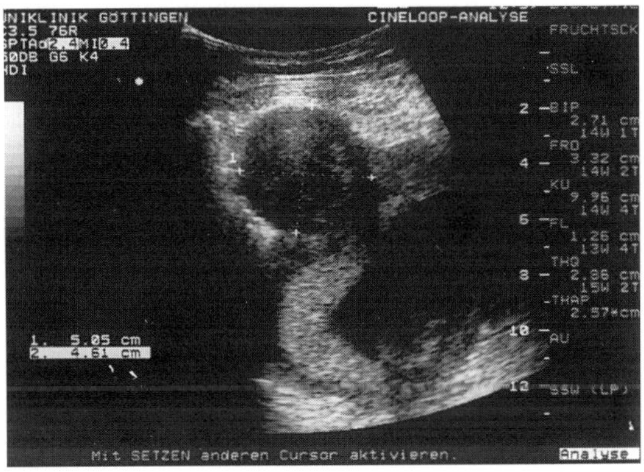

Figure 13 Retroplacental myoma in the 16th gestational week. Hypodensity of the myoma compared to the myometrium. Hypodensity indicates good vascularization.

size of myomas can vary enormously. In very large myomas, transabdominal sonography should be preferred; in very small ones, transvaginal sonography. Myomas measuring 10–15 mm or more can already be localized. Sometimes, myomas are located symmetrically on both sides of the midline. According to Hörmann (cited by Strauss[16]), this would indicate genesis of myomas as a dysraphian disorder leading to inaccurate fusion of Müllerian ducts. The sonographic picture of myomas varies depending on the histological status. Myomas with good vascularization show a more hypoechogenic structure, compared to normal uterine tissue (Figure 13). Homogeneous, hyperechogenic myomas have often undergone regressive changes and have a large amount of connective tissue. Other regressive changes such

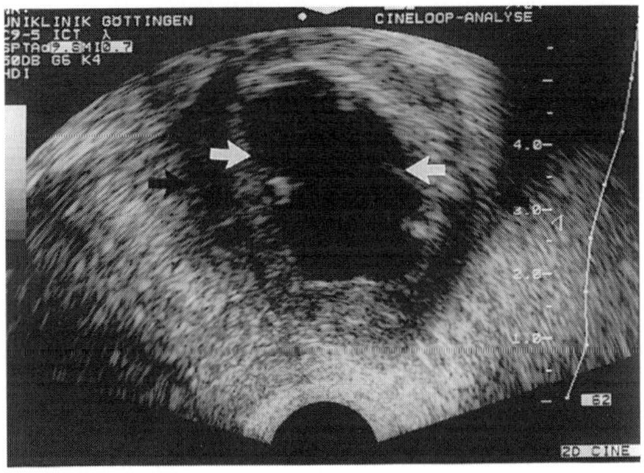

Figure 14 Transverse section showing myoma (black arrows) with central necrosis (white arrows)

as necrosis (Figure 14) and carneous or cystic degeneration can be recognized by the presence of hypoechogenic regions or regions without echogenicity in the myoma. If there is necrosis of the myoma, it can be confounded with an ovarian cyst. Hyalinization and calcification are responsible for bright reflections with partially diffuse shadowing behind. Calcified myomas can therefore impair or disable their delimitation and sonographic localization.

While intramural and submucous myomas can easily be detected by ultrasound, subserous myomas can cause diagnostic problems. Subserous myomas, located in the fundus, can be concealed by intestinal loops, or their cranial delimitation can be difficult to determine. Pedunculated myomas, in particular when they are attached to the posterior wall of the uterus, or intraligamentary myomas cannot be differentiated from solid ovarian tumors for reasons of anatomy and sonomorphology, with one exception: when there is evidence of a pedicle. Pedunculated submucous myomas can lead to ballooning of the corpus uteri or cervix, or, if they are in statu nascendi, can be seen adjacent to the external os of the cervix. Cervical myomas can be confounded with a barrel-shaped carcinoma of the cervix, if there is ballooning of the latter.

If a conservative approach is planned, evaluation of the growth of the myoma is important. As it is not always possible to measure the myoma in the same cross-section when re-examining, it is advantageous for comparative assessment to determine the myoma's volume.

MALIGNANT CHANGES OF THE MYOMETRIUM

Sarcomas of the uterus are relatively rare and account for 1–3% of all malignant tumors of the uterus. Besides irregular genital bleeding, especially in stromal sarcomas, and rapid growth, there are scarcely any clinical symptoms. Whether one is dealing with a myoma or sarcoma in a space-occupying lesion, appearing sonographically as a myoma, can only be proven by histological examination. Nevertheless, there are, similar to macroscopic aspects, sonographic indications for the existence of a sarcoma. If there is evidence of rapid growth of a pre-described myoma in a postmenopausal woman, and in ultrasound an increase of echoless areas as a sign of necrosis, laparotomy should be performed (Figure 15).

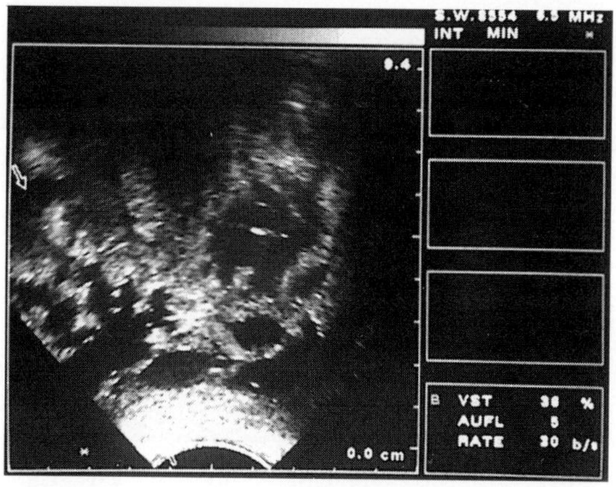

Figure 15 Sarcoma of the uterus with the typical structural signs of heterogeneous necrosis of the tumor

Primary sarcomas in ultrasound examinations appear as poorly outlined masses, partly hyperechogenic, partly irregularly limited and hypoechogenic, or without echogenicity. Differentiation from myomas can be facilitated by the absence of any systematic structure (onion-skin or whirlpool pattern). Differential diagnosis of inhomogeneous, myometrial masses can be myomas undergoing carneous degeneration, with a pool of liquid or bleeding into the myoma. They may resemble sarcomas sonographically. Bleeding can cause a sudden growth of the myoma or of the uterus. If there are myometrial masses, Cacciatore and associates[18] strongly recommend laparotomy, in order to exclude sarcoma.

References

1. Hata, K., Nishingaki, A., Makihara, K., Takaniya, O., Hata, T. and Kitao, M. (1989). Ultrasonic evaluation of the normal uterus in the neonate. *J. Perinat. Med.*, **17**, 313–17
2. Deutinger, J. and Bernaschek, G. (1986). Normgrößen des inneren Genitales bei Mädchen vor und nach der Menarche. *Wiener Klin. Wochensch.*, **98**, 465–8
3. Orsini, L. F., Salardi, S., Pilu, G., Bovicelli, L. and Caccari, E. (1984). Pelvic organs in premenarcheal girls: real-time ultrasonography. *Radiology*, **153**, 113–16
4. Gurr, S., Kobs, K. and Steindel, E. (1986). Ultraschallmessungen des Uterus bei Jugendlichen. *Zent.Bl. Gynkol.*, **108**, 1420–4
5. Platt, J. F., Bree, R. L. and Davidson, D. (1990). Ultrasound of the normal nogravid uterus: correlation with gross and histopathology. *J. Clin. Ultrasound*, **18**, 15–19
6. Bartl, W., Nasr, F. and Bernaschek, G. (1984). Die Beeinflussung zyklusabhängiger Größenveränderungen der Gebärmutter durch Einnahme hormonaler Kontrazeptiva. *Ultraschall*, **5**, 74–6
7. Nasri, M. N., Setchell, M. E. and Chard, R. (1990). Transvaginal ultrasound for diagnosis of uterine malformations. *Br. J. Obstet. Gynaecol.*, **97**, 1043–5
8. Stein, A. L. and March, C. M. (1990). Pregnancy outcome in women with mullerian duct anomalies. *J. Reprod. Med.*, **35**, 411–14
9. Carrington, B. M., Hricak, H., Nurvadin, R. N., Secaf, E., Laros, R. K. and Hill, E. C. (1990). Mullerian duct anomalies: MR imaging evaluation. *Radiology*, **176**, 715–20
10. Rock, J. A. (1992). Surgery for anomalies of the mullerian ducts. In Thompson, J. D. and Rock, J. A. (eds.) *Te Linde's Operative Gynecology*, 7th edn. pp. 603–46. (Philadelphia: J. B. Lippincott)
11. Azziz, R. (1989). Adenomyosis: current perspectives. *Obstet. Gynecol. Clin. North AM.*, **16**, 221–35
12. Fedele, L., Bianchi, S., Dorta, M., Arcaini, L., Zanotti, F. and Carinelli, S. (1992). Transvaginal

ultrasonography in the diagnosis of diffuse adenomyosis. *Fertil. Steril.*, **58**, 94–7
13. Bird, G. C., McElin, T. W. and Manalo-Estrella, P. (1972). The elusive adenomyosis of the uterus – revisited. *Am. J. Obstet. Gynecol.*, **112**, 583–93
14. Walsh, J. W., Taylor, K. J. M. and Rosenfeld, A. T. (1979). Gray scale ultrasonography in the diagnosis of endometriosis and adenomyosis. *Am. J. Radiol.*, **64**, 87–90
15. Bohlmann, M. E., Ensor, R. E. and Sanders, R. C. (1987). Sonographic findings in adenomyosis of the uterus. *Am. J. Radiol.*, **148**, 755–6
16. Strauss, G. (1991). Uterus Körper. In von Psychrembel, W., Strauss, G. and Petri, E. (eds.) *Praktische Gynkologie 5*, revised edn, pp. 179–92. (Berlin, New York: Walter de Gruyter)
17. Merz, E. (1988) Uterustrumoren. In Merz, E. (ed.) *Sonographische Diagnostik in Gynkologie und Geburtshilfe. Lehrbuch und Atlas*, pp. 40–44. (Stuttgart, New York: Georg Thieme Verlag)
18. Cacciatore, B., Lehtovirta, P., Wahlström, T. and Ylostalo, P. (1989). Ultrasound findings in uterine mixed mullerian sarcomas and endometrial stromal sarcomas. *Gynecol. Oncol.*, **35**, 290–3

Uterine leiomyoma: transvaginal color Doppler studies and new aspects of management

8

F. Aleem and M. Predanic

Uterine leiomyomas are benign proliferations of smooth muscle cells and fibrous connective tissue arising from uterine smooth muscle. They are the most common pelvic tumors in women of reproductive age; 20–25% of women have uterine leiomyomas[1]. Leiomyomas are hormone-dependant neoplasms. They arise only during the reproductive years and tend to regress after menopause, implicating estrogen as a growth promotor. Higher concentrations of estrogens[2] and estrogen receptors[3,4] within leiomyomas than in adjacent myometrium were taken as evidence of the hormone-dependance of their growth.

The majority of leiomyomas are asymptomatic. Estimates of the percentage of leiomyomas that are symptomatic range from 10 to 40%. The most common symptom associated with leiomyoma is abnormal bleeding, which typically presents clinically as menorrhagia. Pelvic pain is the second most common symptom, although uterine leiomyomas are probably not directly responsible. Acute pain associated with low-grade fever, localized uterine tenderness and mild peritoneal signs may be observed either with degeneration or, more rarely, with torsion of a pedunculated subserous tumor. Pelvic pressure and lower urinary tract complaints are reported in up to one-third of women undergoing myomectomy[5]. Reproductive disorders, including infertility, recurrent spontaneous abortion and preterm labor have been attributed to uterine leiomyoma.

The diagnosis of uterine leiomyoma can be established with approximately 95% confidence on the basis of physical examination[7]. Leiomyomas are suspected on the basis of bimanual pelvic examination that reveals an enlarged, firm, nontender and irregularly contoured uterus. Leiomyomas of more than 12 weeks' growth – equivalent to the gestational size – can easily be palpated on abdominal examination. Several studies have established the accuracy of radiographic studies, particularly ultrasonography and magnetic resonance imaging, in the diagnosis and measurement of uterine leiomyomas[8–10]. Routine ultrasonographic imaging of leiomyomas allows for accurate assessment of the location, number and size of tumors, differentiation from adnexal masses compromised by uterine size, and documentation of interval growth with serial studies.

ULTRASONOGRAPHY

Uterine leiomyomas may be single or multiple, may range in size from 1 mm to more than 20 cm in diameter, and are surrounded by a pseudocapsule of compressed muscle fibers. Leiomyomas may be located within the uterine wall (intramural) or may protrude into the endometrial cavity (submucous) or from the serosal surface of the uterus (subserosal) (Figure 1). Pedunculated subserosal tumors that outgrow their uterine blood supply and obtain a secondary blood supply from another organ, such as the omentum, are termed parasitic leiomyomas. Leiomyomas located in the lower uterine segment and cervix are associated with a higher frequency of obstructed labor, Cesarean sections and retained placentas[11]. Pedunculated subserosal leiomyomas may extend laterally outward between the folds of the broad ligament (intraligamentary) and simulate adnexal masses.

The most common sonographic appearance of the uterine leiomyomas is of a hypoechoic or heterogeneous uterine mass[8]. When multiple

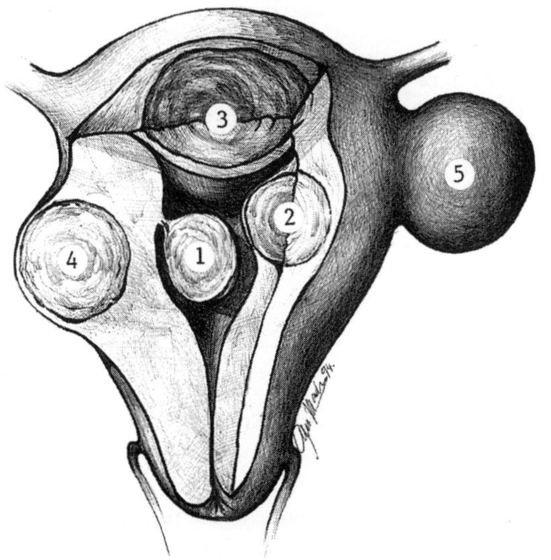

Figure 1 Schematic presentation of uterine leiomyomas and their location: (1) submucous pedunculated; (2) submucous; (3) intramural; (4) partially subserosal and (5) entirely subserosal

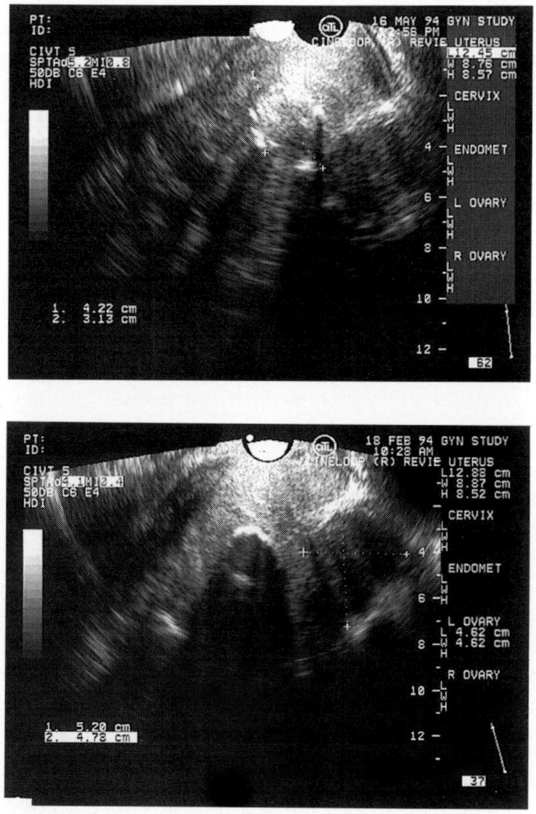

Figure 2 Intramural calcified leiomyoma demonstrated as hyperechogenic ring with thin shadows around the leiomyoma (upper), or as hyperechogenic semi-lunar rim with a large shadow below it (lower)

small leiomyomas are present, sonography may merely show globular uterine enlargement. Submucous or small intramural leiomyomas may be recognized by their distortion of the normally linear central endometrial echo. Occasionally, a large submucous myoma will be seen as a mass within the endometrial cavity, with the endometrial echoes draped over the mass. The sonographic texture of leiomyomas depends on the relative ratio of fibrous tissue to smooth muscle and on the presence and type of degeneration. With a more fibrous component, there is increased echogenicity of the mass. Central ischemia, which is a consequence of tumor enlargement and inadequate blood supply, is usually followed by various stages of degeneration. Therefore, leiomyomas may be minimally echogenic; irregular anechoic areas are seen if cystic degeneration is present[12].

Clusters of high-level echoes with distal acoustic shadowing are quite common with calcified degeneration. Calcifications may vary from a few small foci to a large rim or globular calcification (Figure 2), and are present in approximately 25% of leiomyomas[13]. Carneous degeneration during pregnancy may cause severe pain and appear sonographically as a heterogeneous pattern with cystic spaces within the fibroid[14].

Small leiomyomas can easily be confused with adenomyosis of the uterus. It was reported that this condition can be diagnosed sonographically, because of the thickened, 'Swiss cheese' appearance of the myometrium, caused by areas of hemorrhage and clots within the muscle[12]. However, this image of the adenomyosis can be found only on rare occasions. More common findings for adenomyosis are the presence of an inhomogeneous circumscribed area in the myometrium, with ill-defined margins, and containing anechoic lacunae of varying diameters[9]. This finding can be easily distinguished from the leiomyomas, which are nodular formations with well-defined margins, heterogeneous structure and variable echogenicity.

Table 1 Blood flow visualization rates and hemodynamic characteristics – resistance index (RI), pulsatility index (PI), and peak systolic velocity (Ps) (cm/s) – of the leiomyoma-supplying vessels and main uterine artery

	Uterine artery											
	Control				*Leiomyoma*				*Leiomyoma-supplying vessels*			
Authors	*n*	*PI*	*RI*	*Ps*	*n*	*PI*	*RI*	*Ps*	*Rate* (%)	*PI*	*RI*	*Ps*
Hata *et al.*[17]	8	–	0.94	–	31	–	0.76	–	–	–	–	–
Hata *et al.*[18]	10	–	0.76*	–	21	–	0.68*	–	–	–	–	–
Kurjak *et al.*[19]	60	2.52	0.84	34.1	71†	1.65	0.74	47.1	70	0.89	0.54	–
Kurjak and Zalud[20]	–	–	–	–	231	–	–	–	58	–	0.58	–
Matta *et al.*[21]	–	–	–	–	8	–	0.52	–	100	–	0.48	–

n, number of patients with leiomyomas; rate, blood flow visualization rate; *, arcuate arteries; †, only vascularized leiomyomas

Leiomyomas during pregnancy show rapid growth, obstruction of labor and uterine inversion. However, one half of all leiomyomas detected during pregnancy do not change significantly in size[11]. Growth changes demonstrated by the remainder of leiomyomas depend on their previous size. Small leiomyomas tend to increase in size during the first and second trimesters and decrease in size during the third trimester. Large leiomyomas tend to increase in size only in the first trimester and decrease in size during the second and third trimesters[11].

COLOR DOPPLER STUDIES

Transvaginal color Doppler ultrasound, a new technique, provides accurate information that can be related to the pathophysiological and hemodynamic changes of the pelvic reproductive organs. It can be used to assess leiomyoma vascularity, as well as the physiological and pathophysiological characteristics of uterine artery blood flow[15,16]. The presence and growth of uterine leiomyomas is correlated with the increase of blood flow in the uterine vascular network. A decrease of vascular impedance to blood flow in the main uterine arteries – resistance (RI) or pulsatility (PI) indices – can be found[17–21], as well as an increase in blood flow velocities (Table 1). Decreased vascular resistance to blood flow can be explained by larger concentrations of estrogens and estrogen receptors[2–4] within leiomyomas than in adjacent myometrium, subsequently causing vasodilatation of the uterine vascular network.

The mean RI value of 0.84 for the uterine artery in the control group of patients, obtained from the aforementioned studies (Table 1), was significantly higher than in the group of patients with uterine leiomyomas (RI = 0.67). The mean RI value of 0.53 for the supplying vessels of leiomyomas can be seen, but blood flow visualization rates range from 58 to 100%[19–21]. All uterine leiomyomas should be well vascularized, in comparison to the rest of the normal myometrial tissue, due to their possession of a large number of estrogen receptors. Therefore, discrepencies in reporting the blood flow visualization rates for leiomyomas might be explained by differences in technique and the lack of detailed methodology.

The vascularization of leiomyomas is supported by pre-existing myometrial vessels originating from terminal branches of the uterine artery. A leiomyoma grows centripetally as proliferations of smooth muscle cells and fibrous connective tissue, creating a pseudocapsule of compressed muscle fibers. Therefore, color Doppler demonstrates most of the leiomyometrial blood vessels at its periphery.

We speculated, from our own observations, that blood vessels, displayed as thick vessels encircling the leiomyoma, usually represent dilated veins (Color plate A), whereas blood vessels that 'perforate' the peripheral part of the leiomyoma tissue are usually arteries. Vessel density depends on its location within the leiomyometrial tissue. Peripherally located vessels are dense, because they represent extensions of uterine arcuate and pre-existing myometrial vessels,

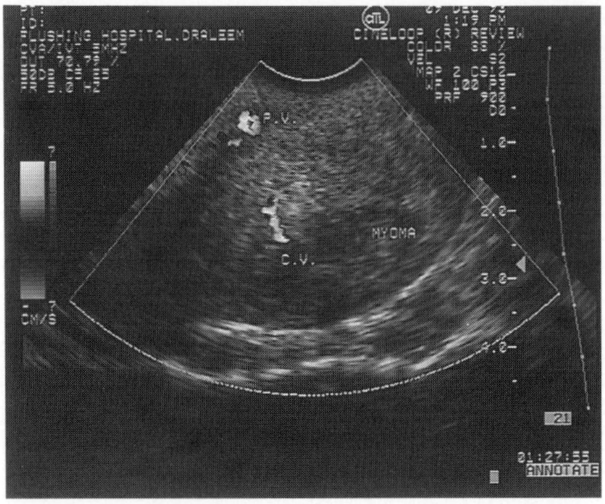

Figure 3 Central vascularity of the leiomyoma (C.V.) with low vascular impedance to blood flow displayed by pulsed Doppler (RI = 0.37; PI = 0.48). P.V., peripheral blood vessels

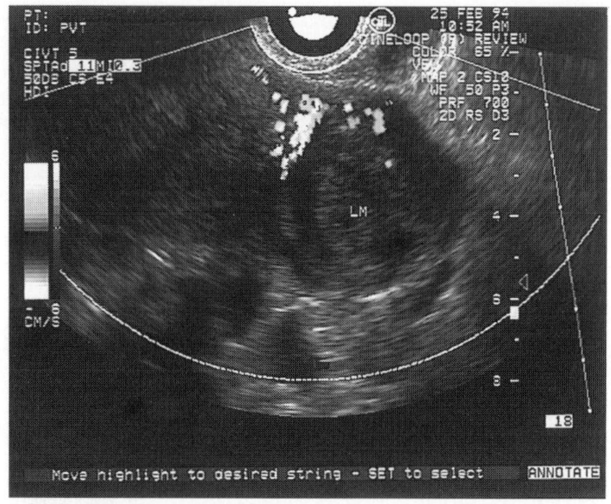

Figure 4 Entirely subserosal leiomyoma with extremely vascularized base (arrow)

while blood vessels demonstrated within the central part are scattered and rarely observed (Figure 3). The presence of blood vessels in the central portion of the leiomyomas is usually correlated with necrotic, degenerative and inflammatory changes. These vessels display lower RI values than do peripherally located vessels, and can sometimes be misinterpreted as malignant neovascularization by the pulsed Doppler signal[19].

Vascular impedance to blood flow in leiomyometrial supplying vessels depends not only on size but also on location within the uterus. In our prospective study, we evaluated the morphology, size, location and vascularity of 42 leiomyomas. Vascular impedance, expressed in terms of RI, PI and peak-systolic velocity, was related to the location of the leiomyomas within the uterus. Leiomyomas were categorized as submucous, intramural, and partially and purely subserosal (located at the surface of the uterine wall) (Figure 4, Color plate B). All leiomyomas were well vascularized peripherally, while central vascularization was found in only four leiomyomas (7.5%). Blood flow characteristics are presented in Table 2.

A significant difference was shown in blood flow characteristics for leiomyoma-supplying vessels between entirely subserosal vs. partially subserosal leiomyomas ($p < 0.001$), and entirely subserosal vs. intramural leiomyomas ($p < 0.001$) (Figures 5, 6 and 7). The lowest RI and PI values for entirely subserosal leiomyomas can be explained by the fact that these leiomyomas are supplied with blood vessels through a very small contact area. These blood vessels, surrounded by loose tissue, are the only source of nourishment and are, therefore, dilated with very low vascular impedance to blood flow.

MANAGEMENT OF LEIOMYOMA AND THE ROLE OF COLOR DOPPLER SONOGRAPHY

Currently available options for treatment of uterine leiomyoma include non-surgical modalities as well as surgical procedures. Non-surgical methods include management and administration of gonadotropic releasing hormone (GnRH) agonists, while surgical methods include either abdominal, laparoscopic or hysteroscopic myomectomy and abdominal or vaginal hysterectomy.

GnRH agonist treatment

Medical therapy may be the best way to treat large submucous leiomyomas and to facilitate hysteroscopic resection; await imminent onset of menopause in the perimenopausal age group;

Table 2 Resistance index (RI), pulsatility index (PI) and peak-systolic velocity (Ps) (cm/s) obtained from leiomyometrial supplying vessels of 53 uterine leiomyomas from different intrauterine locations in 42 patients

		RI		*PI*		*Ps*	
Uterine location	*n*	*Mean*	*SD*	*Mean*	*SD*	*Mean*	*SD*
Submucous	2	0.50	0.01	0.78	0.07	7.5	2.1
Intramural	32	0.59	0.11	1.06	0.31	19.7	12.3
Partially subserosal	10	0.62	0.07	1.22	0.31	23.7	10.1
Entirely subserosal	9	0.43	0.08	0.58	0.17	29.0	16.1
Total	53	0.57	0.11	0.99	0.33	20.8	13.1

n, number of leiomyomas

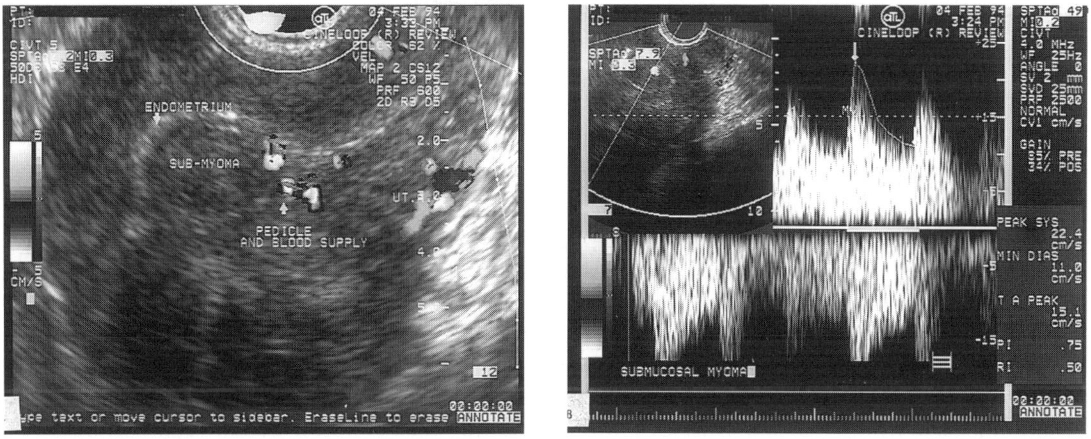

Figure 5 Submucous leiomyoma (left) endometrium surrounds leiomyoma and increased vascularity at the base of the leiomyoma can be noted; (right) pulsed Doppler signal obtained from the vessel located at the base of the submucous leiomyoma

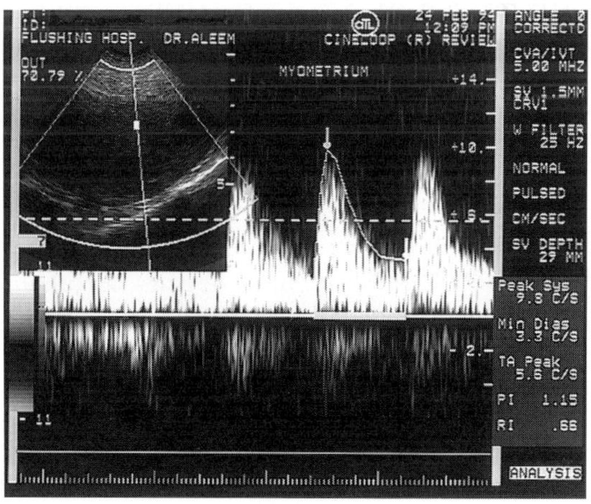

Figure 6 Pulsed Doppler sonogram of an intramural leiomyoma with moderate vascular impedance to blood flow (RI = 0.66; PI = 1.15)

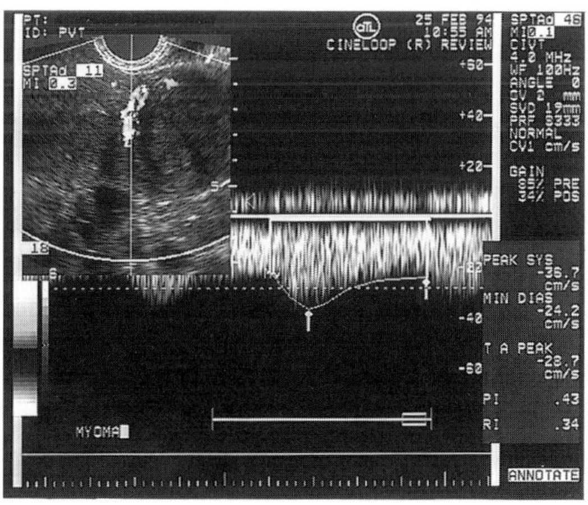

Figure 7 Very low vascular impedance to blood flow (RI = 0.34; PI = 0.43) obtained from the vessel located in the pedicle of a subserous leiomyoma

decrease leiomyoma size; and reduce symptoms while awaiting surgery. Synthetic GnRH agonists inhibit estrogen production, causing the uterine mass to shrink. Filicori and co-workers[4] first reported treatment of a patient with a uterine leiomyoma and anemia with a GnRH agonist. Numerous studies have since been performed and have confirmed the ability of GnRH agonists to induce uterine and leiomyoma shrinkage and menstrual suppression. Friedman[22] reported reduction of uterine volume in women treated with GnRH agonist for 3–6 months by a mean of 40–50%, and this decrease in uterine size was usually maximal by 12 weeks of treatment. However, approximately 20% of women had a decrease in uterine volume of up to 50%, 50% experienced a moderate volume reduction (26–50%), 25% had a decrease of 0–25% and 5% actually experienced an increase of 0.1–25% in uterine volume[23]. GnRH agonist treatment is no guarantee of continued protection after treatment is stopped. Fibroids usually return to their original size within 4 months[24].

The first reported Doppler study of uterine arteries in leiomyomas under GnRH agonist therapy was performed by Matta and associates in 1988[21]. Their study, which was performed with only eight patients, demonstrated significant increases in vascular resistance of uterine vessels after 4 months of GnRH agonist therapy. Uterine vascularity was assessed in this study by measuring the RI in the uterine and major leiomyoma arteries. The pretreatment RI value of the uterine artery (mean RI = 0.52) and leiomyoma artery (mean RI = 0.48) was significantly increased after treatment (mean RI values of 0.92 and 0.91, respectively). The authors concluded that a decrease in uterine volume under GnRH agonist therapy was a consequence of decreased uterine vascularity.

Recently, Reinsch and colleagues[25] assessed the effects of RU 486 (mifepristone, a synthetic steroid with both antiprogesterone and antiglucocorticoid activities) and leuprolide acetate on uterine artery blood flow of 14 patients. Both groups showed an increase in RI values of uterine arteries and a decrease in uterine volume at 3 months of therapy. Resistance index increased by 2–51% in those patients receiving RU 486, and by

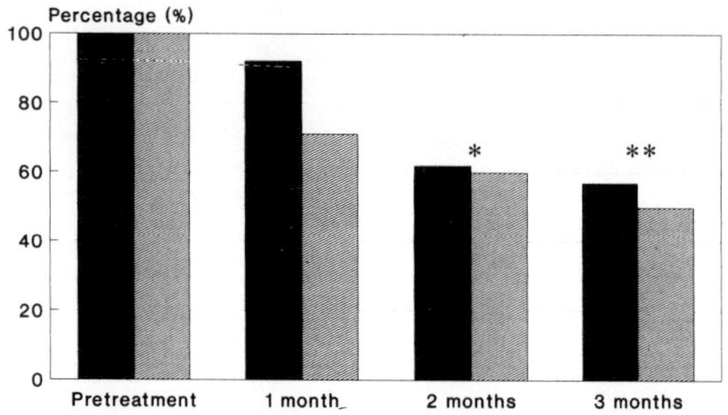

Figure 8 Reduction in the volume of the uterus (black bars) and leiomyoma (hatched bars) after one dose (1 month), two doses (2 months) and three doses (3 months) of GnRH agonist – leuprolide acetate depot. *, $p<0.05$; **, $p<0.001$ (Student's *t*-test)

8–39% for those receiving leuprolide acetate. The authors concluded that an increase in the RI with GnRH agonist was probably caused by the hypoestrogenic effect, while the reduction in blood flow with RU 486 was mediated by another mechanism.

In a prospective study, we evaluated 23 women with clinically diagnosed uterine leiomyomas, who received GnRH agonist therapy for 3 months. Pretreatment measurements of total uterine volume, individual leiomyoma volume, RI, PI and peak-systolic velocity were compared with post-treatment values 4, 8 and 12 weeks after GnRH agonist therapy (3.75 mg leuprolide acetate, depot suspension, TAP Pharmaceuticals, Chicago, USA). Total uterine volume and individual volume for any identifiable leiomyoma were calculated after measurement of the three largest dimensions (D) of each, and by using the formula for a prolate ellipsoid ($D_1 \times D_2 \times D_3 \times 0.52$). Transvaginal color and pulsed Doppler sonography (at 5 MHz) were used to demonstrate and assess the blood-flow characteristics for main uterine and leiomyoma-supplying arteries. The color Doppler pulsed repetition frequency range of 400–900 Hz and pulsed Doppler sample volume from a width of 1 mm were used. Statistical analysis was by Student's *t*-test.

Table 3 shows a summary of the results obtained prior to and after the GnRH agonist therapy in 23 patients with uterine leiomyomas. A significant difference in reduction of total uterine volume, individual leiomyoma volume, increase

Table 3 Summary of results obtained prior to and after 3 months of GnRH agonist therapy (leuprolide acetate depot) in 23 patients with uterine leiomyomas

	Pretreatment		*Post-treatment*	
	Mean	*SD*	*Mean*	*(SD)*
Total uterine volume (cm^3)	202	79	117	31*
Individual leiomyoma volume (cm^3)	74	42	33	25*
Uterine artery RI	0.73	0.07	0.87	0.06*
Uterine artery PI	1.48	0.40	2.31	0.49*
Uterine artery Ps	43.4	12.7	37.6	11.2
Leiomyoma artery RI	0.55	0.10	0.71	0.09*
Leiomyoma artery PI	0.96	0.29	1.48	0.61*
Leiomyoma artery Ps (cm/s)	20.8	10.3	15.4	4.9

*, $p<0.001$ (Student's t-test), pretreatment vs. post-treatment values; RI, resistance index; PI, pulsatility index; Ps, peak-systolic velocity

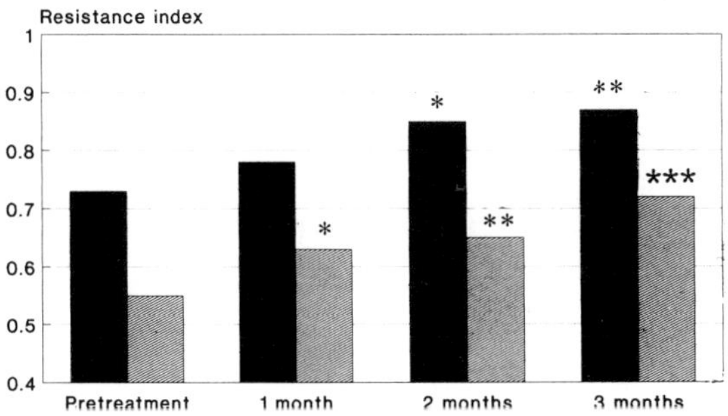

Figure 9 Increase in mean resistance index for uterine artery (black bars) and leiomyometrial arteries (hatched bars) after one dose (1 month), two doses (2 months) and three doses (3 months) of GnRH agonist – leuprolide acetate depot. *, $p<0.05$; **, $p<0.01$; ***, $p<0.001$ (Student's t test)

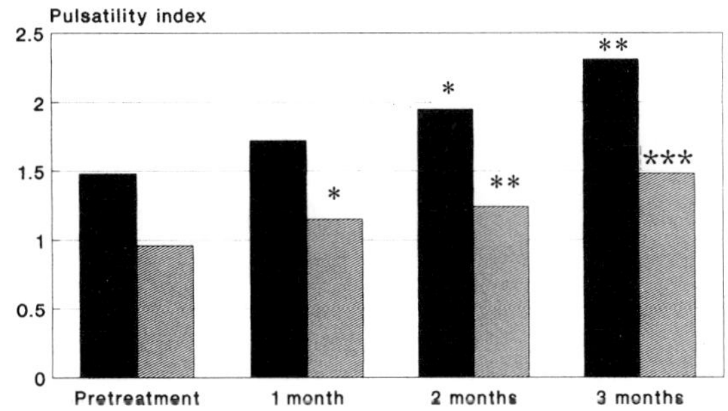

Figure 10 Increase in mean pulsatility index for uterine artery (black bars) and leiomyometrial arteries (hatched bars) after one dose (1 month), two doses (2 months) and three doses (3 months) of GnRH agonist – leuprolide acetate depot. *, $p<0.05$; **, $p<0.01$; ***$p<0.001$ (Student's t test)

of uterine artery RI and PI values and leiomyoma artery RI and PI values was found in this study (Table 3). There was no statistically significant difference in peak-systolic velocity between the uterine and leiomyoma arteries.

A statistically significant reduction of total uterine and leiomyoma volumes was obtained after a second dose of leuprolide acetate ($p<0.05$), which correlated with a significant drop in serum estradiol levels. The reduction of uterine and leiomyoma volumes was even more pronounced after a third dose of luprolide acetate ($p<0.001$) (Figure 8). This result is in agreement with a previously published report by Friedman and co-workers[26]. Our results showed a reduction of the mean uterine artery volume by 42% after the third dose of GnRH agonist treatment. This reduction of uterine volume correlated with the uterine volume reduction range of 34–61% demonstrated in 12 reported studies after 3–6 months of GnRH agonist therapy (buserelin, leuprolide, goserelin, nafarelin, G-Trp6 or D-His6-Pro9)[27].

A significant increase in vascular impedance to blood flow (RI and PI values) for the uterine artery was also found after a second dose of GnRH agonist ($p<0.05$). However, a significant difference of RI and PI values for leiomyoma arteries was observed after the first leuprolide acetate dose ($p<0.05$) (Figures 9 and 10), and it was increased further after the second ($p<0.01$) and third doses ($p<0.001$). A significant increase of RI and PI values for leiomyoma arteries, after the first dose, can be explained by the fact that the blood flow of leiomyomas is moderated by the presence of a higher percentage of estrogen receptors than is found in the rest of myometrial tissue. Deprivation of estrogen with GnRH therapy will immediately influence the reduction of leiomyometrial blood flow, while the normal myometrial vascularity, represented by the uterine artery, will respond with a slower rate of reduction.

Surgical methods

Surgical therapy usually involves abdominal, laparoscopic or hysteroscopic myomectomy or abdominal or vaginal hysterectomy. The primary advantage of myomectomy is uterine conservation with preservation of fertility. Hysterectomy is the definitive treatment for uterine leiomyoma in symptomatic women who have completed childbearing. The risk of mortality associated with hysterectomy performed for benign indications is approximately one per 1000 procedures[28,29].

However, endoscopic resection of leiomyomas, as a new modality, has recently been introduced. Laparoscopic resection of subserosal and intramural leiomyomas has been reported[30], but the benefit of laparoscopic removal of myomas has not been established. Recent cases have documented potential complications, including uterine dehiscence[31].

In comparison with these surgical methods, alternative treatment of uterine leiomyomas with laparoscopic myolysis by Nd:YAG laser showed promising results, although in a limited study[32]. The bare laser fiber was laparoscopically introduced into the leiomyoma. During application of laser energy, the leiomyoma was repeatedly drilled to degrade the leiomyometrial stroma, denature protein, destroy vascularity and substantially shrink fibroids. The distance between each hole was about 5–7 mm, desiccating a cone of vasculature approximately 3–5 mm in diameter around each puncture point. Repeated puncturing effectively destroys the leiomyoma. Hormonal and sexual function is preserved, because the uterus is left intact. Follow-up after 6 months with ultrasonography showed that the echostructure of the coagulated leiomyoma was so similar to the normal myometrium that it could only be distinguished by experienced echographers. Long-term follow-up of seven patients, who had open surgery, showed no regrowth of the leiomyoma, while histological study proved the complete devascularization of the leiomyometrial tissue with subsequent necrosis[32].

Our current pilot study is to evaluate the size, vascularity and degenerative changes following the electrocoagulation and destruction of leiomyometrial vasculature through the laparoscope. Color Doppler sonography was used to demonstrate and locate the leiomyoma blood vessels. Accurate placement of bipolar needles directing coagulation to the vascular area, vs. blind coagulation of the whole leiomyoma, may improve the success of the therapy, as well as reduce the duration of the procedure.

We compared the amount of blood flow and shrinkage of the leiomyomas after the bipolar electrocoagulation therapy, where color Doppler had been used as guidance for destruction of the leiomyoma vascular pedicle, and where coagulation of the whole leiomyoma had been performed with no color Doppler guidance. We noted that in the group where color Doppler was not used prior to surgery, leiomyoma shrinkage was less and supplying blood vessels were more frequent than in the group where color Doppler was used before surgery (Color plate C).

These preliminary results emphasize the value of color Doppler, not only for the accurate assessment of leiomyoma growth, but also for preoperative planning for either open surgery or endoscopic management.

References

1. Vollenhoven, B. J., Lawrence, A. S. and Healy, D. L. (1990). Uterine fibroids: a clinical review. *Br. J. Obstet. Gynaecol.*, **97**, 285–98
2. Wilson, E. A., Yang, F. and Rees, E. D. (1980). Estradiol and progesterone binding in uterine leiomyomata and in normal uterine tissues. *Obstet. Gynecol.*, **55**, 20–4
3. Solues, M. R. and McCarty, K. S. Jr (1982). Leimyomas: steroid receptor content. Variations within normal menstrual cycle. *Am. J. Obstet. Gynecol.*, **143**, 6–11
4. Filicori, M., Hall, D. A., Loughlin, J. S., Rivier, J., Vale, W. and Crowley, W. F. Jr. (1983). A conservative approach to the management of uterine leiomyoma: pituitary desensitization by a luteinizing hormone-releasing hormone analogue. *Am. J. Obstet. Gynecol.*, **147**, 726–7
5. Buttram, V. C. Jr and Reiter, R. C. (1981). Uterine leiomyomata: etiology, symptomatology, and management. *Fertil. Steril.*, **36**, 433–45
6. Cramer, S. F. and Patel, D. (1990). The frequency of uterine leiomyomas. *Am. J. Clin. Pathol.*, **94**, 435–8
7. Gambone, J. C., Reiter, R. C., Lench, J. B. and Moore, J. G. (1990). The impact of a quality assurance process on the frequency and confirmation rate of hysterectomy. *Am. J. Obstet. Gynecol.*, **163**, 545–50
8. Karasick, S., Lev-Toaff, A. S. and Toaff, M. E. (1992). Imaging of uterine leiomyomas. *Am. J. Roentgenol.*, **158**, 799–805
9. Fedele, L., Bianchi, S., Dorta, M., Zanotti, F., Brioschi, D. and Carinelli, S. (1992). Transvaginal ultrasonography in the differential diagnosis of adenomyoma versus leiomyoma. *Am. J. Obstet. Gynecol.*, **167**, 603–6
10. Hricak, H. (1986). MRI of the female pelvis: a review. *Am. J. Roentgenol.*, **146**, 1115–22
11. Lev-Toaff, A. S., Coleman, B. G., Arger, P. H., Mintz, M. C., Arenson, R. L. and Toaff, M. E. (1987). Leiomyomas in pregnancy: sonographic study. *Radiology*, **164**, 375–80
12. Kurjak, A. and Zalud, I. (1991). Uterine masses. In Kurjak, A. (ed.) *Transvaginal Color Doppler*, pp. 93–102. (Carnforth, UK: Parthenon Publishing)
13. Gross, B. H., Silver, T. M. and Jaffe, N. H. (1983). Sonographic features of uterine leiomyomas: analysis of 41 proven cases. *J. Ultrasound Med.*, **2**, 401–5
14. Altchek, A. (1991). Management of uterine leiomyomata. In Altchek, A. and Deligdisch, L. (eds.) *The Uterus*, pp. 344–65. (New York: Springer-Verlag)
15. Hata, T., Hata, K., Senoch, D., Makihara, K., Aoki, S., Takamiya, O., Kitao, M. and Umaki, K. (1990). Transvaginal Doppler flow mapping. *Gynecol. Obstet. Invest.*, **27**, 217–18
16. Kurjak, A., Shalan, H., Kupesic, S., Predanic, M., Zalud, I., Breyer, B. and Jukic, S. (1993). Transvaginal color Doppler sonography in the assessment of pelvic tumor vascularity. *Ultrasound Obstet. Gynecol.*, **3**, 137–54
17. Hata, T., Hata, K., Senoh, D., Makihara, K., Aoki, S., Takamiya, O. and Kitao, M. (1989). Doppler ultrasound assessment of tumor vascularity in gynecologic disorders. *J. Ultrasound Med.*, **8**, 309–14
18. Hata, K., Makihara, K., Hata, T., Takahashi, K. and Kitao, M. (1991). Transvaginal color Doppler imaging for hemodynamic assessment of reproductive tract tumors. *Int. J. Gynecol. Obstet.*, **36**, 301–8
19. Kurjak, A., Kupesic-Urek, S. and Miric, D. (1992). The assessment of benign uterine tumor vascularization by transvaginal color Doppler. *Ultrasound Med. Biol.*, **18**, 645–9
20. Kurjak, A. and Zalud, I. (1991). The characterization of uterine tumors by transvaginal color Doppler. *Ultrasound Obstet. Gynecol.*, **1**, 50–2
21. Matta, W. H. M., Stabile, I., Shaw, R. W. and Campbell, S. (1988). Doppler assessment of uterine blood flow changes in patients with fibroids receiving the gonadotropin-releasing hormone agonist Buserelin. *Fertil. Steril.*, **49**, 1083–5
22. Friedman, A. J. (1993). Treatment of uterine myomas with GnRH agonists. *Semin. Reprod. Endocrinol.*, **11**, 154–61
23. Friedman, A. J., Daly, M., Juneau-Norcross, M. and Rein, M. S. (1992). Predictors of uterine volume reduction in women with myomas treated with a gonadotropin releasing-hormone agonist. *Fertil. Steril.*, **58**, 413–15
24. Donnez, J. and Nisolle, M. (1992). Hysteroscopic surgery. *Curr. Opin. Obstet. Gynecol.*, **4**, 439–55
25. Reinsch, R. C., Murphy, A. A., Morales, A. J. and Yen, S. S. C. (1994). The effects of RU 486 and leuprolide acetate on uterine artery blood flow in the fibroid uterus: a prospective, randomized study. *Am. J. Obstet. Gynecol.*, **170**, 1623–8
26. Friedman, A. J., Barbieri, R. L., Doubilet, P. M., Fine, C. and Schiff, I. (1988). A randomized, double-blind trial of gonadotropin-releasing hormone agonist (leuprolide) with or without medroxyprogesterone acetate in the treatment of leiomyomata uteri. *Fertil. Steril.*, **49**, 404–9
27. Stewart, E. A. and Friedman, A. J. (1992). Steroidal treatment of myomas: preoperative and long-term medical therapy. *Semin. Reprod. Endocri-*

nol., **10**, 344–56

28. Dicker, R. C., Greenspan, J. R., Strauss, L. T., Cowart, M. R., Scally, M. J. and Peterson, H. B. (1982). Complications of abdominal and vaginal hysterectomy among women of reproductive age in the United States. *Am. J. Obstet. Gynecol.*, **144**, 841–8
29. Wingo, P. A., Huezo, C. M., Rubin, G. L., Ory, H. W. and Peterson, H. B. (1985). The mortality risk associated with hysterectomy. *Am. J. Obstet. Gynecol.*, **152**, 803–8
30. Garry, R., Erian, J. and Grochmal, S. A. (1991). A multi-centre collaborative study into the treatment of menorrhagia by Nd-YAG laser ablation of the endometrium. *Br. J. Obstet. Gynaecol.*, **98**, 357–62
31. Harris, W. J. (1992). Uterine dehiscence following laparoscopic myomectomy. *Obstet. Gynecol.*, **80**, 545–6
32. Nisolle, M., Smets, M., Malvaux, V., Anaf, V. and Donnez, J. (1993). Laparoscopic myolysis with the Nd:YAG laser. *J. Gynecol. Surg.*, **9**, 95–9

The development and the structure of the uterus

9

Lj. Kostović-Knežević and Đ. Grbeša

THE DEVELOPMENT OF THE UTERUS

Prenatal development

Embryos of both sexes develop in an identical fashion prior to the 8th week (the indifferent stage). Only thereafter do anatomical and physiological development diverge to result in the formation of the male or female phenotype[1]. During the indifferent stage of sexual differentiation, the primordial genital tract of both sexes consists of paired undifferentiated gonads, mesonephric tubules, a dual duct system (mesonephric–Wolffian and paramesonephric–Müllerian ducts) and an unpaired urogenital sinus (the ventral portion of the embryonic cloaca). All these primordia are composed of an epithelial element surrounded by mesenchyme[2].

Within the mesonephros, tubules are connected with a longitudinal mesonephric (Wolffian) duct that extends caudally to the primitive urogenital sinus. It is the excretory duct for the mesonephric kidney. Normal phenotypic sexual development is determined by the presence (in males) or the absence (in females) of specific hormonal signals at the critical time in embryonic development. In the female, there is the tendency of genital structures to develop into the female type in the absence of specific masculinizing influences. The absence of testosterone inhibits the development of the mesonephric ducts. They either disappear or persist in remnant form. The absence of anti-Müllerian hormone (AMH), also known as Müllerian inhibiting substance (MIS) allows the development of the paramesonephric ducts[3]. They develop into the uterine tubes and uterus, and contribute to the development of the vagina.

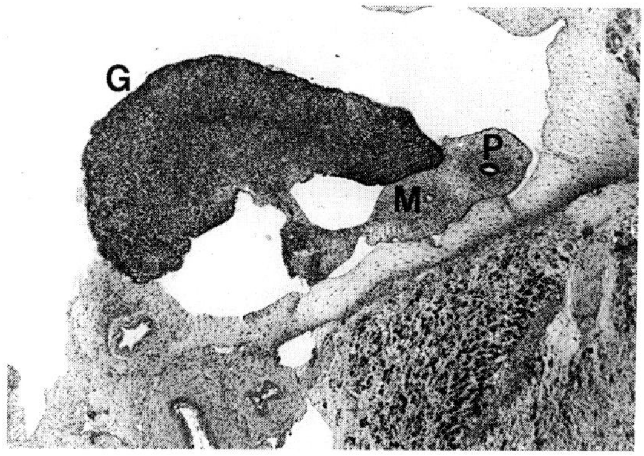

Figure 1 Development of the genital ducts in the 8-week human embryo (crown–rump length 25 mm). G, gonad; M, mesonephric duct; P, paramesonephric duct (×42)

The first description of the genesis of the paramesonephric duct was made by von Müller, in 1830[4]. The paramesonephric (Müllerian) ducts appear in both sexes, one on each side of the body, but attain complete development only in the female. In the human, the paramesonephric duct appears in embryos of nearly 6 weeks (10 mm) as a groove in the thickened celomic epithelium on the surface of the urogenital ridge. The cranial end of the groove remains open, and later persists as the abdominal ostium of the uterine tube. The caudal tip of the invagination forms a solid bud, which burrows in the mesenchyme lateral to and parallel with the mesonephric duct (Figure 1). As the bud increases in length, a lumen appears in its upper part and gradually extends towards the growing tip.

Early development and growth of the paramesonephric duct occur without direct stimulation, i.e. with neither gonadotropins nor the ovary. The outgrowing paramesonephric duct has been

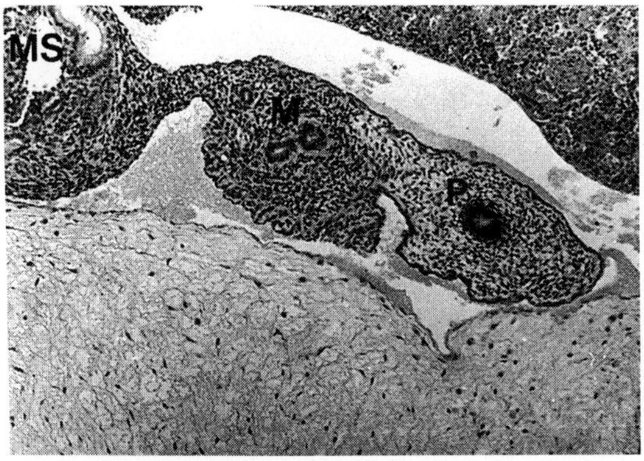

Figure 2 The genital ducts and the mesonephros of the 8-week embryo. P, paramesonephric duct; M, mesonephric duct; MS, mesonephros (× 192)

investigated at the light- and electron microscopic level[5,6]. The mesonephric and paramesonephric ducts are separated by mesenchyme. Both ducts are enclosed by basal lamina of their own (Figure 2). The paramesonephric ducts are simple, straight tubes lined with a single-layered epithelium consisting of cells ranging from squamous to cylindrical. As they grow, the epithelium becomes taller, with basally situated nuclei. Parallel to the epithelial growth, mesenchymal cells are arranged in concentric layers around the ducts. Further differentiation of the ducts depends on mesenchymal–epithelial interaction.

The mesenchyme is the target and mediator of morphogenetic action by hormones[7]. The periductal stroma differentiates during the 7th and 8th weeks. Among the mesenchymal cells that concentrate around the duct, some light cells appear. They are epithelioid cells originating from the celomic epithelium. During the 8th and 9th weeks, the number of light stromal cells decreases and most cells degenerate. By the 12th week, only a small number of light cells are left. Meanwhile, the amount of dark fusiform cells of mesonephric origin increases in the periductal stroma. The duct grows rapidly. The light stromal cells should be regarded as a separate cellular system, different from the dark, fusiform cells. The light, epithelial cells secrete the extracellular material. The dark cells are supposed to be involved in the breakdown of the epithelio–stromal interface[6].

The epithelial cells of the paramesonephric duct form a columnar epithelium. After the duct's differentiation completed during the 7th week of development, the distance between the two ducts is short. It then decreases in the caudal direction, so that the paramesonephric duct contacts the lateral face of the mesonephric duct. In the segment of the terminal bud and its tip there exists only one common basal lamina for mesonephric and paramesonephric ducts. Their cells are in close contact. They are described as 'intermediate cells' or 'transitional cell types', i.e. cells that are not clearly recognizable as mesonephric or paramesonephric cells. Desmosomes among the mesonephric cells are frequent; contacts among paramesonephric cells can also be found. These cells are interdigitated among each other. They form finger-like cytoplasmic protrusions which are connected by desmosomes. At the tip of the terminal bud, a cluster of cells lies adjacent to the mesonephric duct. The caudal part of the mesonephric duct shows a one-layered epithelium enclosed by a continuous basal lamina[4].

In the embryo of 9 weeks, the caudal blind tip of the paramesonephric duct reaches the pelvic area, and crosses in front of the mesonephric duct to its medial side. It continues to grow in a caudo–medial direction till it fuses with the duct of the opposite side in the midline, dorsocranially to the urogenital sinus[7–9] (Figure 3). The paramesonephric ducts fuse into a solid core of cells, the uterovaginal primordium (Figure 4).

In the embryo of 10 weeks (32 mm), the fused portion of the paramesonephric ducts ends blindly and projects into the dorsal wall of the urogenital sinus. Below the caudal tip of the uterovaginal primordium and above the dorsal wall of the urogenital sinus, a collection of paramesonephric cells forms the Müllerian tubercle (sinus tubercle).

In the absence of androgenic stimulation, the mesonephric ducts begin to regress and fragment. The paramesonephric ducts persist and grow. Near the cloaca, the two urogenital ridges swing toward the midplane and fuse to the so-called genital cord. The progressively elongating paramesonephric ducts, originally lateral in position, are brought side-by-side in the midplane (Figure 5). When the urogenital ridges are crowded laterally by the enlarging suprarenal glands and

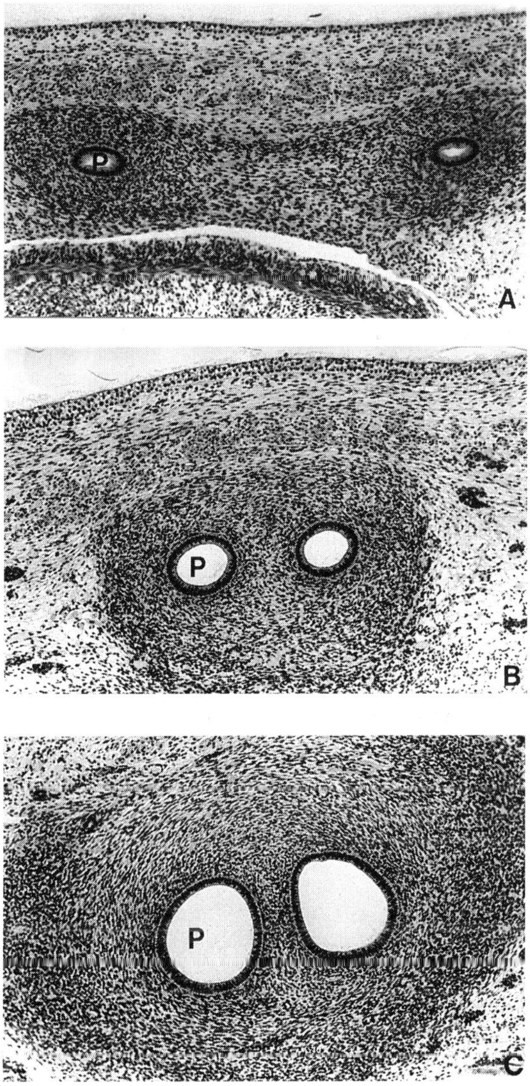

Figure 3 Development (A–C) of the uterine primordium during the 3rd lunar month. In the caudal region, the paramesonephric ducts (P) cross ventral to the mesonephric ducts and come together in the midline (× 172)

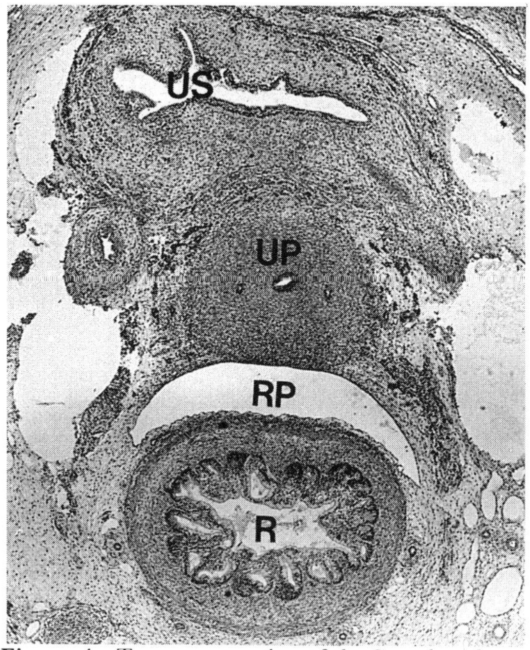

Figure 4 Transverse section of the 8-week embryo. US, early urogenital sinus; UP, uterine primordium; RP, rectouterine pouch; R, rectum (× 50)

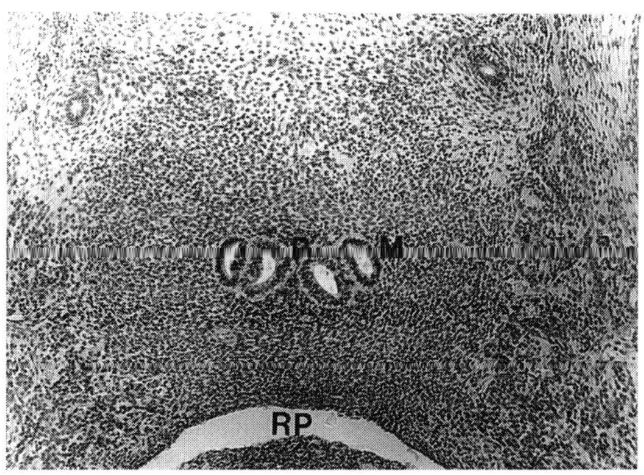

Figure 5 Development of the genital ducts. P, paramesonephric duct; M, mesonephric duct; RP, rectouterine pouch (× 162)

permanent kidneys, each paramesonephric duct in its course makes two bends, which establish three definitive regions:

(1) A cranial, longitudinal portion (uterine tube);

(2) A middle, transverse portion (uterine fundus and corpus); and

(3) A caudal longitudinal portion, which fuses with the other portion to produce a common tube (uterine cervix and vagina).

The cranial or unfused portion of each paramesonephric duct becomes the uterine tube. Its open end develops fimbriae[9]. However, the adequate development and fusion of the paramesonephric

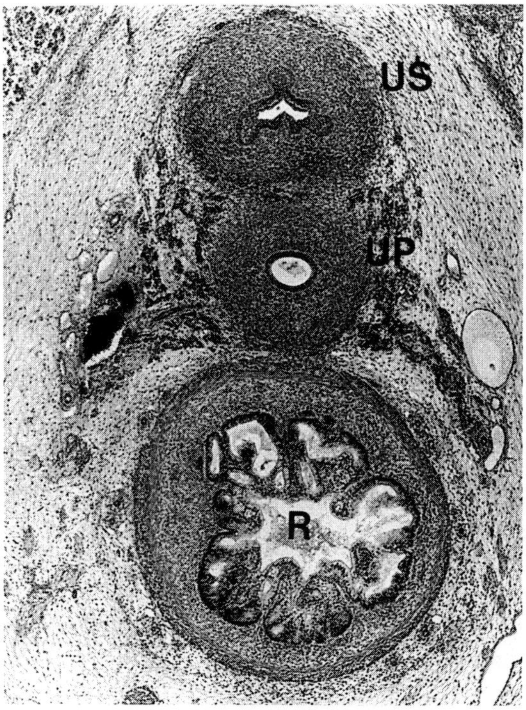

Figure 6 Transverse section of the 8-week embryo, showing the fused paramesonephric ducts and the development of the uterine primordium (UP). US, urogenital sinus; R, rectum (× 56)

ducts, the reabsorption of the septum between them and the formation of a normal definitive uterus is induced by the laterally situated mesonephric ducts. They act as guide elements for the paramesonephric ducts[3] (Figure 5).

The fusion of the paramesonephric ducts is at first partial and there is a temporary septum between the two lumina. This septum disappears at the 56-mm stage, so that a single cavity, the uterovaginal canal, is formed. This canal is lined with cuboidal epithelium. The cranial point of fusion marks the future site of the fundus of the uterus. In primates, complete caudal union of paramesonephric ducts produces a common uterus and a common vagina, but only in the highest primates does the union reach its fullest expression[9]. As the result of complete fusion of the paramesonephric ducts, the uterus is pear-shaped, with a single lumen, and is called a simplex uterus (Figure 6).

The caudal end of the uterus opens into the vagina in the form of an unpaired neck or cervix. The most caudal portion of the fused paramesonephric ducts (mesodermal elements) is nearest the Müllerian tubercle and the urogenital sinus (endodermal elements). The uterovaginal canal and cells derived from it give rise to the epithelial lining of the uterus and to the upper part of the vagina. Proliferation of the tip of the uterovaginal canal results in the formation of a solid vaginal cord that increases the distance between the uterovaginal lumen and the urogenital sinus. Laterally, the mesonephric ducts enter the urogenital sinus. During female development, the mouth of the mesonephric duct is transformed into an epithelial pocket carrying the degenerating mesonephric duct at its cranial end. The bilateral pockets proliferate and form two solid epithelial ('sino-vaginal') bulbs, extending as dorsolateral projections from the urogenital sinus[10]. The sino-vaginal bulbs fuse with the vaginal cord and a vaginal plate arises. The Müllerian tubercle incorporates itself in the vaginal plate and disappears.

The vaginal plate is formed from the endodermal epithelium of the urogenital sinus and from the caudal end of the uterovaginal primordium. The vaginal plate is recognizable in the fetus at 60–75 mm, and is fully developed in the fetus at 150 mm. It becomes canalized through breakdown of central cells, but not until the 162-mm stage[8], although some authors have described it as early as during the 12th week of development[11].

There are major changes in the vagina during the 5th lunar month. Thus, by mid-pregnancy, the fusion of the paramesonephric ducts is completed and the vaginal lumen is present. This cavitation allows the paramesonephric cells to line the primitive vaginal cavity with a cuboidal or paramesonephric epithelium. The lumen of the vagina is separated from the urogenital sinus by the hymenal membrane until late fetal life.

The developmental processes involved in morphogenesis of the female genital tract are similar in most vertebrate species. The mesenchyme induces and specifies epithelial differentiation. Epithelial–mesenchymal interactions are phenomena initiated in the embryo and perpetuated throughout reproductive life. Autoradiographic analysis of the developing urogenital sinus and paramesonephric ducts of embryonic mice indicates that nuclear estrogen receptors are restricted to the mesenchyme surrounding the paramesonephric and mesonephric ducts. Mesenchyme induces and directs the expression of epithelial development, including cytodifferentiation and function[2,12,13].

The vaginal epithelium is derived from the endoderm of the urogenital sinus. The outer fibromuscular wall is derived from the uterovaginal primordium of mesodermal origin. Near the external cervix is the junction between the mesodermal epithelium of the uterus and the endodermal epithelium of the vagina[14]. Later, the endodermal epithelium of the urogenital sinus invades and replaces the paramesonephric epithelium. The vagina becomes lined by a stratified squamous epithelium.

Differentiation of the uterus starts with that of the uterine tube. The junction between them soon becomes distinguishable by the increase in the uterine diameter. At about 9.5 weeks, the fetal uterus begins to differentiate into the corpus and the cervix. They are both initially the same length, but the cervix gradually reaches two-thirds of the total length at birth. The uterine portion of the uterovaginal canal is not completely separated from the vaginal portion. Demarcation between the uterus and vagina takes place later, at the end of the 3rd month, when the fornices appear[7].

Embryogenesis takes place in a milieu of steroidal and non-steroidal hormones derived from the placenta, the maternal circulation and the fetal adrenal glands. It is not known whether any of these substances influences female phenotypic differentiation or early development. Estrogens and progesterone are involved in the growth and maturation of the female urogenital tract during the later part of fetal development.

The upper portion of the uterovaginal primordium gives rise to the epithelium and glands of the uterus. The endometrial stroma and myometrium are derived from the adjacent mesenchyme (Figure 7).

The uterine mucosa differentiates during the second half of fetal development. Prior to the 5th month of gestation, a single layer of columnar epithelium lines the uterine cavity. There are no glands and the subepithelial stroma is not different in appearance from the mesenchyme that will become the myometrium. Towards the end of the 6th month, the epithelium forms pouches of cells which grow into the underlying mesenchyme. These structures will become the endometrial glands. Glands first appear in the cervical part at 17 weeks. About 2 weeks later, they also appear in the corpus.

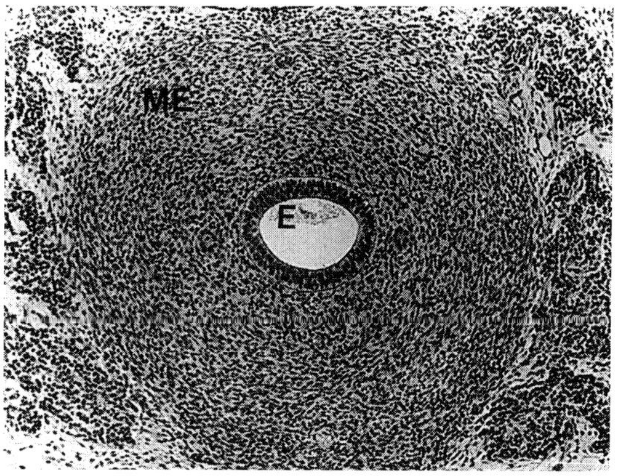

Figure 7 The uterine primordium during the 8th week of development. E, epithelium; ME, mesenchyme (× 175)

At approximately 20 weeks, mesenchyme surrounding paramesonephric ducts condenses. Smooth muscle cells appear in the wall of the uterus and form the early muscular layer of the uterus, the myometrium and its peritoneal covering, the perimetrium. The development of the muscular layer during the second half of gestation changes the shape of the fetal uterus. The growing muscular layer of the upper part of the corpus participates in the formation of the fundus. The caudal two-thirds of the uterus has become a narrow neck or isthmus leading into the cervix. The corpus of the developing uterus is short and bulbous.

By the 7th month, the endometrial glands are evident and the endometrium of the fetal uterus responds to the steroid hormones produced by the placenta. The proliferating glandular epithelium resembles that found in adult endometrium during the proliferative stage of the menstrual cycle. During the 8th month of gestation, the glands begin to coil and the stroma becomes edematous[15].

During the third trimester of development,

mucinous cells appear in the cervix. They are rarely seen in the endometrium at birth[7].

Up to the 32nd week, the fetal ovary secretes no estrogen. The estrogenic and progesteronic activity of any steroid hormones which enter the fetal body is reduced as a result of metabolic degradation within the fetal liver. It is only from the 32nd week that in normal pregnancies the estrogen acts on the fetal uterine cervix. This action consists of hyperplasia of the endocervical epithelium and its emergence towards the exocervix[16].

In late fetal life there is a high production of placental estrogen. There is a corresponding increase in the growth of the fetal uterus as a result of the hormonal stimulation. The thickness of the endometrium and the myometrium increases with fetal age. The thickness of the myometrium increases rapidly from 0.13 mm in the 12th week to 0.65 mm in the 36th week of gestation. The thickness of the endometrium changes slowly from 0.15 mm in the 12th week to 0.40 mm in the 36th week of gestation[17]. By the 9th month, the fetal endometrium is hypertrophic. The blood vessels are congested and the coiled glands actively secrete.

Postnatal development

The neonatal endometrium resembles the adult endometrium. It has features of both proliferative and secretory endometrium. Hyperemia, glandular tortuosity and thicker endometrium are evident. Secretory changes and decidual reaction are frequently seen. The uterine cavity is often filled with large amounts of blood, epithelial remnants and denuded stroma, as a consequence of maternal hormonal stimulation[18].

In the full-term neonate, the serum concentration of estrogen drops rapidly after birth. Enlargement of the uterus is the effect of maternal estrogen. The neonatal uterus is larger and thicker than the prepubertal uterus as a result of stimulation from maternal hormones. The uterus is tubular or spade-shaped, with the anterior–posterior diameter of the cervix equal to or greater than the anterior–posterior diameter of the fundus. The length of the uterus shows a significant correlation with birth weight[18] and it ranges from 2.3 to 4.6 cm, with a mean of 3.4 cm. Two-thirds is the cervix, and only one-third is the corpus. The uterus is approximately 0.6–0.9 cm longer than the normal prepubertal uterus. The endometrial thickness is 0.2–0.4 cm.

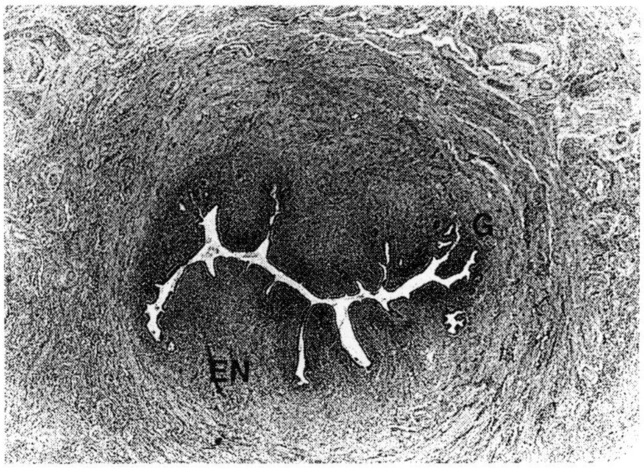

Figure 8 Transverse section of the infant uterus. EN, thin endometrium with dense stroma; G, low, tubulous uterine glands (× 36)

Morphometric studies of the uterus between the 1st and 11th year of life show a longitudinal growth of the uterus of about 10 mm[19]. The infant's cervical mucous glands and uterine endometrium are in an active, stimulated state.

During infancy and childhood, the corpus remains smaller than the cervix. The mean uterine length is 2.5 cm and mean width is 1 cm. The endometrial glands elongate, reaching the basal portion of the endometrium. The endometrium is thin and has a dense stroma (Figure 8). Endocervical glands become inactive, low and tubulous, and are lined with cuboidal epithelium. The mean uterine length in prepubertal girls over the age of 1 year is 2.8 cm[20]. From 2 to 7 years of age, the mean uterine length is approximately 3.3 cm and increases to 4.2 cm at 11 years, 6.2 cm at 13 years and 7 cm at 17 years[21,22] (Table 1). The cervix occupies two-thirds to five-sixths of the total uterine length and the corpus is half the diameter of the cervix[20]. It is tubular, with similar cervical and fundal diameters (0.7–0.8 cm)[21].

Up to 7 years of age, uterine size is not influenced by age. The uterus has an 'inverse' pear-shaped morphology, because the prepubertal uterus is thicker in the cervix than in the corpus, while the opposite is true in the postpubertal uterus.

Table 1 Morphometric studies of the human uterus between the 1st and 17th year of life

	Age (years)					
	1	*2–7*	*11*	*13*	*17*	*Authors*
Uterine length (cm)	2.8	3.3	4.2	6.2	7	Orsini *et al.* (1984)[21]; Ivarsson *et al.* (1983)[22]
Uterine volume (cm^3)		0.9			53	Schaller (1989)[19]
Cervix (% of total uterine length)	65–80	50		40	40	Sample *et al.* (1977)[20]

From late childhood until menarche, the rate of uterine growth surpasses that of any other part of the female genital tract. This growth occurs primarily in the corpus and predominantly in width and thickness[20]. The uterus gradually reaches its typical adult pear-shaped morphology in older girls[21].

From 7 years onward, there is a measurable age-related increase in uterine diameters and volume. Uterine volume increases from a mean of 0.9 cm^3 at 7 years to 53 cm^3 at 17 years (Table 1). During the 12th to 14th years, there is an accelerated growth amounting in total to 20–30 mm. The longitudinal growth, as well as the distance between portio and fundus, correlate with the girl's body weight and height. The growth in width correlates with the girl's age[19].

After puberty, the corpus of the uterus becomes larger than the cervix. The cervix decreases from 50% of total uterine length at 7 years to 40% at 13–17 years of age[22] (Table 1). This growth is the result of ovarian steroids that act upon the endometrium and the myometrium. The endometrium proliferates and the endometrial glands produce abundant mucous secretions.

Development of the genital ligaments

The ligaments of the genital organs are derivatives of the peritoneum. In the female at 6 weeks of development, the mesonephroi and gonads arise retroperitoneally and bulge into the celom carrying a fold of peritoneum that surrounds them[23]. In the region where the uterovaginal canal develops into the uterus, the mesonephroi and their mesenteries connect the developing uterus with the walls of the pelvic cavity.

In the early fetal period (9–10 weeks) the pelvic cavity is filled with undifferentiated mesenchyme. Between the 11th and 12th weeks, it is replaced by loose connective tissue containing abundant collagenous fibers[24,25]. As the mesonephroi degenerate, a fibrous sheet remains, covered by the peritoneum. It becomes the broad ligament that connects the uterine corpus with the lateral walls and floor of the pelvic cavity. This ligament and the uterus separate the uterorectal (Douglas) and uterovesical pouches of the pelvic cavity. The dorsal and ventral uterine walls are covered by dense connective tissue. The uterorectal ligament increases or decreases in size in relation to the size of the uterus. Ventrally, loose connective tissue is interposed between the bladder and the cervix of the uterus[24,25].

In 16–18 weeks of development, the connective tissue condenses. Between the 19th and 28th weeks, its differentiation has proceeded, and within the pelvic cavity, lobules of adipose tissue have formed. The uterine corpus and cervix are still situated in one plane. Because of the angle between the uterine cervix and the vagina, an anteversion is already visible.

As the ovaries increase, they sag into the body cavity and pull with them the broad ligament. In the female, the inguinal ligament of the mesonephros is embedded in the broad ligament. When the ovaries move caudally and laterally, the inguinal ligament is bent into an angular form. Cranial to the bend, it becomes the round ligament of the ovary and caudal to it, the round ligament of the uterus. The caudal end of the uterine round ligament is embedded in the connective tissue of the labium majus[23].

Abnormal development of the uterus and vagina

The following is an embryological classification of congenital anomalies and disorders of development of the uterus and vagina[26,27].

(1) Agenesis or hypoplasia of the urogenital ridge; there will be an absence of kidney, functioning ovary and the uterine tube, and hemiuterus and hemivagina of the same side;

(2) Mesonephric anomalies with an absence of an opening in the urogenital sinus; there will usually be a uterine anomaly, because of the absence of the inductor function of the mesonephric duct;

(3) Problems of vertical fusion, due to an abnormality in the fusion of the downgrowing paramesonephric ducts with the upgrowing derivative from the urogenital sinus; these may cause a transverse vaginal septum;

(4) Problems of lateral fusion or resorption of the septum, in which duplication abnormalities occur[26]; these problems may involve all or a part of the paired paramesonephric ducts; and

(5) Isolated Müllerian anomalies; there is a proposed classification of the Müllerian anomalies[27]:

Class I (segmental Müllerian agenesis or hypoplasia): vaginal, cervical, fundal, tubal, and combined anomalies. These malformations will most frequently be represented by some form of vaginal malformation (vaginal agenesis), combined with a cervical and/or fundal anomaly. Most often, the uterus is absent or is present only as a rudimentary muscular bud. The atresia of the uterine cervix is the failure of canalization of the cervical segment. This malformation divides the uterine lumen from the vagina. Atresia or agenesis of the vagina develops as failure of the vaginal plate to canalize (vaginal atresia) or failure of the vaginal anlage to form (vaginal agenesis).

Class II (the unicornuate uterus): with or without a rudimentary horn. In this group of anomalies, less commonly, one paramesonephric duct may be partially atretic. The abnormal shape and reduced volume of the uterus are associated with an increased incidence of premature delivery. The reported spontaneous abortion rates vary from 15% to 75%.

Class III (the didelphys uterus): complete failure of the ducts to fuse, leading to the formation of a double uterus with a duplication of the cervix and the vagina. These malformations are frequently associated with premature delivery.

Class IV (the bicornuate uterus): complete, partial, or arcuate. The bicornuate uterus is a more extensive failure of fusion and it is associated with a 20% incidence of premature delivery. The incidence of abortion is increased. The arcuate uterus most closely resembles a 'mild' form of bicornuate uterus. In this malformation, a minor lack of fusion of the ducts leads to a depressed fundus.

Class V (the septate uterus): complete, or incomplete. When fusion of the paired paramesonephric ducts is completed, but the septum between the ductal lumina fails to break down, a septum of variable dimensions may result. Of pregnancies associated with a complete septum, 88% ended in abortion, as did 70% associated with the incomplete form[27].

The frequency of uterine anomalies in a normal fertile population is 3%. The most common malformation is the septate uterus (90%), followed by the bicornuate (5%) and didelphys uterus (5%)[28].

Patients with uterine malformations have high rates of reproductive losses and preterm deliveries. The best fetal survival rates are in the bicornis–bicollis (71%), didelphys (72%), unicornis (71%) and subseptus uterus (69%) groups. The poorest results are obtained in the bicornuate (40%) and arcuate uterus groups (45%)[29].

Incomplete fusion of the paramesonephric ducts may also occur as one component of multiple malformation syndromes, some of which are genetic in origin[30–32]. Primary infertility is also connected with malformation of the uterus. Women with a unicornuate uterus have the highest incidence (15%) of primary infertility[33].

THE STRUCTURE OF THE UTERUS

The uterus is the part of the female reproductive tract situated between the two layers of the broad ligament. It is divided into two major parts, the body (corpus) and the cervix, which are separated by a narrow portion, the isthmus. The body is the rostral expanded part of the uterus. The upper part of the body, from which the oviduct extends, is called the fundus.

The uterus is a highly muscular organ formed by three layers: the endometrium, a glandular mucosa, which has a distinctive vascular supply; the myometrium, a thick tunic of smooth muscle cells; and the outer perimetrium, formed by the serosa (connective tissue and mesothelium), which covers the fundus and much of the posterior part of the uterus, or adventitia (connective tissue), which covers the rest of the free surface of the uterus. The uterus in the non-pregnant condition is 6.5 cm long, 3.5 cm wide and 2.5 cm thick.

The blood supply to the uterus comes primarily from the uterine artery. This vessel approaches the lateral border of the uterus at the level of the isthmus. It continues as a highly tortuous vessel along the lateral border of the uterus, giving branches to both the anterior and posterior surfaces on its way to an anastomosis with the ovarian artery, with which it forms a vascular arch. Some branches of the uterine artery, the arcuate arteries, situated in the middle layer of the myometrium (stratum vasculare), give rise to the small branches situated in the endometrium (see below). The arteries of all three uterine layers are of the muscular type and have an unusually thick tunica media.

The endometrium

The endometrium in menstruating women is composed of two distinct tissue compartments: the upper transient functionalis (stratum functionale), which at the end of each cycle undergoes degeneration and is shed; and the deep germinal basalis (stratum basale), which persists from cycle to cycle[34].

The transient functionalis is subdivided into the stratum compactum, containing the necks of the uterine glands, and the underlying stratum spongiosum, which contains the bodies of the uterine glands (Figure 9). The functionalis has a cyclicity, and during pregnancy, it becomes a part

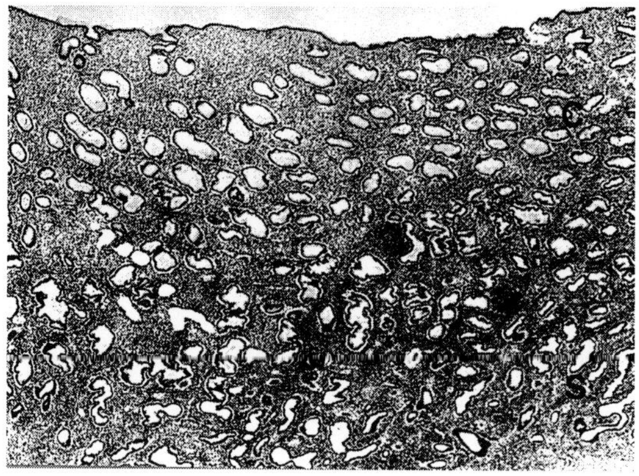

Figure 9 The transient functionalis of the endometrium. C, stratum compactum; S, stratum spongiosum (× 38)

of the maternal placenta. The germinal basalis (stratum basale) is a relatively thin, deep layer in contact with the myometrium. The basalis serves to regenerate the desquamated functionalis during the proliferative phase of the cycle.

Structural and functional changes of the endometrium are dependent on the hormones secreted by the ovaries. The main functions of the endometrium are preparation for implantation of a fertilized ovum, participation in implantation and formation of the maternal portion of the placenta.

The blood supply of the endometrium has a special importance for the mechanisms of menstruation and placentation. The branches of the myometrial stratum vasculare (arcuate arteries) give rise to radial arterioles, which enter the basalis. During their short passage through the basalis, the radial arterioles branch into several basal or straight arterioles, which supply blood to the basalis. On leaving the basalis, the radial arterioles become helical and are referred to as coiled arterioles (Figure 10). These run parallel to the uterine glands, providing a capillary network to supply blood to the stratum spongiosum, and terminate in a subepithelial stratum compactum. Some of these capillaries fuse to form spaces called connecting lacunae[35,36]. From these lacunae and the capillary network, venous blood is collected in the thin-walled collecting lacunae. These carry blood toward the endometrial veins and these drain into the arcuate vein.

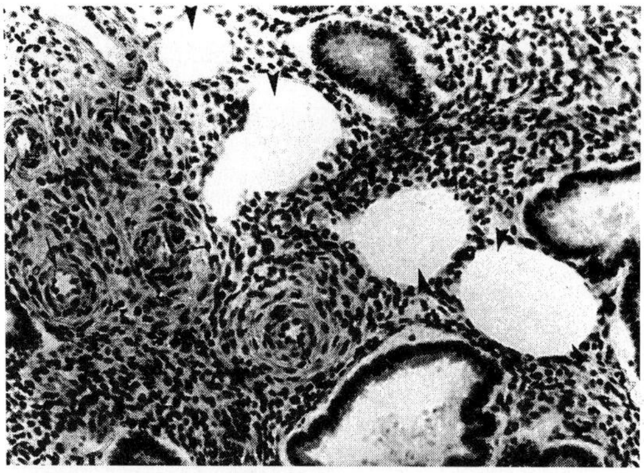

Figure 10 Late secretory phase. Endometrium with coiled arterioles (arrows) and edema in the stroma (arrowheads) (× 178)

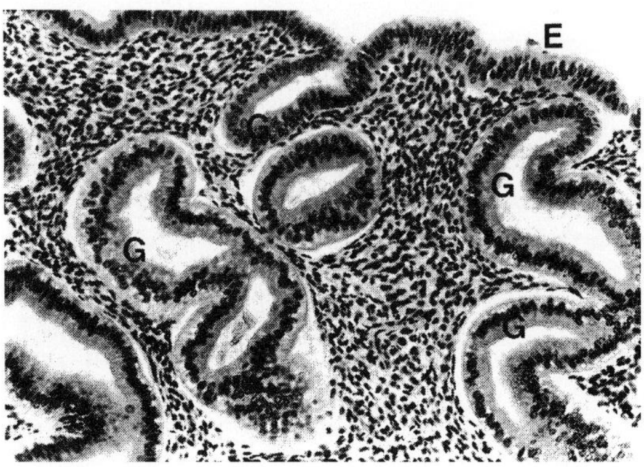

Figure 11 The surface columnar epithelium (E), by invagination, forms numerous tubular uterine glands (G) (× 186)

Coiled arterioles are hormone-sensitive and degenerate and regenerate during each cycle. In pregnancy, the coiled arterioles become placental arteries. Radial and basal arterioles do not react to hormonal changes.

The surface epithelium of the endometrium is simple columnar, composed of a combination of ciliated and secretory cells. The surface-invaginated epithelium forms numerous tubular uterine glands that extend into a thick lamina propria, called the endometrial stroma (Figure 11). The glands are simple tubular, but they may show some bifurcation in the basalis adjacent to the myometrium. They occasionally penetrate among the muscle bundles of the myometrium. The endometrial stroma has irregularly stellate cells, their long processes in contact and adherent to a framework of reticular fibers. Included are lymphoid cells and endometrial granulocytes[37].

The surface epithelium lining the uterine lumen is fused by tight junctions in the lateral cell membranes near the apical pole. These junctions prevent movement of some molecules and serve to isolate the contents of the epithelial lumen from surrounding tissue, as has been shown by experiments[38]. Morphological and morphometric studies have shown that tight junctions between luminal epithelial cells of the uterus change during the menstrual cycle, as well as at the implantation period and during pregnancy[39,40]. Tight junctions play an important role in regulating the flow of fluids to maintain differential microenvironments inside the lumen of the uterus. The changes in the tight junction structure of the uterine epithelial cells may contribute to successful implantation by regulating the uterine luminal contents[41,42].

Cyclic changes in the endometrium

During a normal menstrual cycle, the endometrium passes through a sequence of continous morphological and functional changes under the direct influence of ovarian hormones. Structural and ultrastructural variations occur in the epithelial, stromal and vascular components of the endometrium. These changes in the normal menstrual cycle are so characteristic and well known that they represent a useful model for evaluating and timing ovulation as well as the day of the menstrual cycle or the week of pregnancy that an endometrial biopsy was taken.

Histological dating is carried out using the criteria of Noyes and colleagues[43] and modifications of these[44]. Some other authors have produced additional qualitative and quantitative structural and ultrastructural modifications respecting biological variations[45–51] and hormonal therapy[52–54].

Immunohistochemical studies using qualitative and quantitative receptor assays have enabled the localization and distribution of estrogen and progesterone receptors to be examined in the epithelial and stromal cells of the endometrium. The data from immunohistochemical investigations are a valuable complement to histological and cytological parameters, showing changes in the distribution of estrogen and progesterone receptors during the normal menstrual cycle[55–59] as well as in pathological conditions (endometrial cancer and endometriosis)[60–64].

The endometrial changes, for the convenience of description, are divided into three main phases: the proliferative (follicular) phase, the secretory (luteal) phase and the menstrual phase. Two minor phases, the premenstrual and postmenstrual phase, are also recognized. It must be noted that structural changes that occur during the menstrual cycle are gradual. The division of the phases represents a very helpful model in the clinical investigation of causes of infertility, dysfunction of the ovaries or disorders of menstruation.

Proliferative phase The phase begins at the end of menstrual flow. Mitoses are numerous in the epithelium and in the stroma on the stratum basale. Cellular proliferation continues during the entire proliferative phase, and mitoses are present in the cells of the surface epithelium and in the glands. At the end of the proliferative phase, the glands are straight, and glycogen accumulates within the cells. The coiled arterioles are elongated and start to convolute.

Secretory phase This phase starts after ovulation under the hormonal influence of the corpus luteum. The glands become tortuous with a dilated lumen (Figure 12). Secretion in the glandular epithelium is very active, and the epithelium shows a characteristic cytomorphological structure[44]. The stroma becomes very edematous and loose textured (Figure 10). The stromal cells undergo hypertrophy, and therefore the stroma becomes very thick (5–7 mm) at the end of this phase. The elongation and convolution of the coiled arterioles continue and they extend into the superficial portion of the endometrium.

Menstrual phase At the end of the secretory phase, the walls of the coiled arterioles constrict, so that the ischemia and subsequent necrosis take place in the superficial endometrial zone. The glands stop secreting. Many leukocytes are found at this time in the stroma. After vasoconstriction, the arterioles open up. There is subsequent extravasation

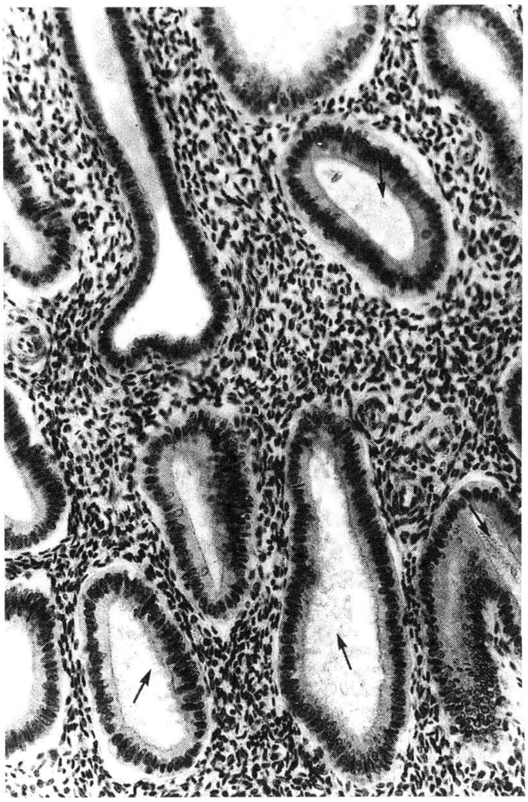

Figure 12 Secretory phase. The glands are active, containing secretory products in the lumen (arrows) (×278)

of the blood through the damaged vessels, and bleeding begins. The entire compacta and a considerable portion of the spongiosa are detached.

The deep ends of glands located in the germinal basalis are the regenerating zone for the new glands and surface epithelium. The superficial circulation is restored too, as well as the stroma, and the proliferative activity of the new cycle begins.

During pregnancy, under hormonal influence, structural and functional differentiation continues, producing decidualization – a change in which stromal cells transform into large, polygonal decidual cells. These cells are arranged in mosaic fashion in the zona compacta.

After the menopause, the endometrium atrophies and becomes thin. The openings of the glands may become partly obliterated and form small cysts.

The myometrium

The myometrium is the thickest tunic of the uterus. It is composed of bundles of smooth muscle cells separated by considerable connective tissue. The bundles of smooth muscle cells form four layers that are not well defined.

Beneath the endometrium is a thin layer of smooth muscle cells called the stratum submucosum. The muscle cells are predominantly longitudinal. The next layer is the thickest, called the stratum vasculare, because it contains many large blood and lymphatic vessels. This layer has circular and oblique muscle bundles. The succeeding stratum supravasculare has muscle bundles that are mainly circular and longitudinal. The outermost stratum subserosum is a thin longitudinal muscle layer. The two most superficial layers send muscular bundles into the wall of the oviduct and into the broad and round ligaments.

The connective tissue is situated between the muscular bundles and consists of collagen fibers, fibroblasts, macrophages and undifferentiated cells. Elastic fibers are present only in the peripheral layers of the myometrium.

In the non-pregnant uterus, the muscle cells are about 0.25 mm in length. During pregnancy, they increase in size and may reach a length of 5 mm by the end of gestation. The maintenance of normal size and cytological characteristics of uterine smooth muscle cells depends on estrogen production. In the absence of estrogen, smooth muscle cells atrophy[65].

The changes in the myometrial thickness during the menstrual cycle have been well documented by means of sagittal magnetic resonance imaging[66]. The average rate of increase in myometrial thickness was 3.2% per day during the proliferative phase and 1.8% per day during the secretory phase of the menstrual cycle; a statistically significant difference.

The myometrium during pregnancy

During pregnancy, the myometrium undergoes a period of great growth. The growth is due to both hypertrophy and hyperplasia (an increase in the number of the cells). At this period, many smooth muscle cells have the ultrastructural characteristics of protein-secreting cells. There is evidence that smooth muscle cells as well as connective tissue fibroblasts of the pregnant uterus are associated with the synthesis and secretion of connective tissue proteins, especially collagen fibrils[65–70]. There is a marked increase in the total amount of uterine collagen.

During the last 20 weeks of gestation, the uterus ceases to increase in weight and the myometrium becomes progressively thinner. Toward the end of pregnancy, gap junctions arise among smooth muscle cells and increase in number. The gap junction is a type of intercellular junction where the adjacent cell membranes, although closely apposed, are separated by a 2-nm space (the 'gap'). The gap between membranes is bridged at intervals by structures (which are recognizable after special preparation) called connexons. A connexon is an assembly of six protein subunits. When connexons in the plasma membranes of two adjacent cells are aligned, they form a direct channel of communication between the two cells[71]. It has been demonstrated that gap junctions are capable of allowing transfer of chemicals and mediators of hormonal stimulation such as cyclic AMP between cells[72]. Gap junctions are important in smooth muscle cells, because they provide for the intercellular flow of potassium ions, responsible for muscle activation. This junctional coupling results in synchronous muscular activity that facilitates delivery. Formation and regulation of myometrial gap junctions as affected by ovarian steroids and the increased production of prostaglandins at term[73–77].

The cervix

As has been noted above, the cervix (collum) is the caudal, cylindric part of the uterus. The cervical mucosa (endocervix) is 3–5 mm thick with a different structure from that of the corpus uteri. The cervical mucosa does not desquamate during menstruation, and during the menstrual cycle undergoes small structural variations. It lacks coiled arterioles. Under the cervical mucosa is situated the fibromuscular layer. High-resolution magnetic resonance images have demonstrated the correlation between the histological and immunohistological zonal anatomy of the cervix[78].

The cervical mucosa forms branching folds called plicae palmatae, which have longitudinal, transverse and oblique arrangements. The surface epithelium of the cervical mucosa consists of tall columnar mucus-secreting cells, with some ciliated cells. The outer surface of the portio vaginalis is covered with stratified squamous epithelium. The mucosa contains numerous large glands, which differ from those of the corpus and isthmus. They are branched, and contain mucus-secreting columnar cells, similar to those of the surface epithelium. These cells produce cervical mucus. Some of the glands become occluded, and the accumulation of secreted mucus transforms these glands into cysts that may be of large diameter. In pregnancy, the cervical glands enlarge, proliferate and abundantly accumulate mucus. The biophysical properties of the mucus are determined by the influence of estrogens and progesterones on the secretory cells. The mucus is composed of glycoprotein rich in carbohydrates. It is a colloid with rheological characteristics of visco-elasticity[34].

Under the cervical mucosa is a thick wall composed predominantly of dense connective tissue: collagenous and elastic fibers with fibroblasts. The smooth muscle cells form only 15% of the tissue. In the portio vaginalis, the smooth muscle cells are absent.

In the very late stage of pregnancy, the intercellular matrix of the connective tissue of the cervical wall begins to change, resulting in the softening of the cervix. At parturition, the hormonally regulated activation of collagenase causes enzymatic breakdown of collagen fibrils[34]. These changes facilitate dilatation of the cervix.

ACKNOWLEDGEMENT

The authors express their gratitude to the Department of Histology and Embryology, School of Medicine, University of Zagreb, for collections of human embryos, fetuses and adult uteri used for research and documentation.

References

1. Wilson, J. D., Griffin, E., Leshin, M. and George, F. W. (1981). Role of gonadal hormones in development of the sexual phenotypes. *Hum. Genet.*, **58**, 78–84
2. Cunha, G. R., Shannon, J. M., Neubauer, B. L., Sawyer, L. M., Fujii, H., Taguchi, O. and Chung, L. W. K. (1981). Mesenchymal–epithelial interactions in sex differentiation. *Hum. Genet.*, **58**, 68–77
3. Acién, P. (1992). Embryological observations on the female genital tract. *Hum. Reprod.*, **7**, 437–45
4. Dohr, G. and Tarmann, T. (1984). Contacts between Wolffian and Müllerian cells at the tip of the outgrowing Müllerian duct in rat embryos. *Acta Anat.*, **120**, 123–8
5. Didier, E. (1973). Recherches sur la morphogénèse du canal de Müller chez les Oiseaux. *Roux Arch. Entw. Mech. Org.*, **172**, 271–302
6. Wartenberg, H. (1985). Morphological studies on the role of the periductal stroma in the regression of the human male Müllerian duct. *Anat. Embryol. (Berl.).*, **171**, 311–23
7. Byskov, A. G. and Hoyer, P. E. (1988). Embryology of mammalian gonads and ducts. In Knobil, E. and Neill, J. D. (eds.) *The Physiology of Reproduction*, vol. I, pp. 265–302. (New York: Raven Press)
8. Hamilton, W. J., Boyd, J. D. and Mossman, H. W. (1947). The urogenital system. In Hamilton, W. J., Boyd, J. D. and Mossman, H. W. (eds.) *Human Embryology*, pp. 193–225. (Cambridge: W. Heffer & Sons)
9. Arey, L. B. (1965). The genital system. In Arey, L. B. (ed.) *Developmental Anatomy*, pp. 315–41. (Philadelphia: W. B. Saunders)
10. Bok, G. and Drews, U. (1983). The role of the Wolffian ducts in the formation of the sinus vagina: an organ culture study. *J. Embryol. Exp. Morphol.*, **73**, 275–95
11. Terruhn, V. (1980). A study of impression moulds of the genital tract of female fetuses. *Arch. Gynecol.*, **229**, 207–17
12. Cunha, G. R. (1975). The dual origin of vaginal epithelium. *Am. J. Anat.*, **143**, 387–92
13. Cunha, G. R., Chung, L. W. K., Shannon, J. M., Taguchi, O. and Fujii, H. (1983). Hormone-induced morphogenesis and growth: role of mesenchymal–epithelial interactions. *Recent Prog. Horm. Res.*, **39**, 559–98
14. Burnett, L. S. (1988). Embryology. In Jones III, H.

W., Colston Wentz, A. and Burnett, L. S. (eds.) *Novak's Textbook of Gynecology*, pp. 89–100. (Baltimore: Williams & Wilkins)
15. Brenner, R. M. and Maslar, I. A. (1988). The primate oviduct and endometrium. In Knobil, E. and Neill, J. D. (eds.) *The Physiology of Reproduction*, vol. I, pp. 303–29. (New York: Raven Press)
16. Minh, H. N., Smadja, A. and Remotti, G. (1993). Hormones et embryogenese du col uterin. *Rev. Fr. Gynecol. Obstet.*, **88**, 151–5
17. Mukerje, B. (1980). Measurements of the human fetal uterus and ovary. *Acta Obstet. Gynecol. Scand.*, **59**, 549–50
18. Nussbaum, A. R., Saunders, R. C. and Douglas, J. M. (1986). Neonatal uterine morphology as seen on real-time US. *Radiology*, **160**, 641–3
19. Schaller, A. (1989). Zur Frage des Uteruswachstums während der endometriuminaktiven Phase. *Wien. Klin. Wochenschr.*, **101**, 352–9
20. Sample, W. F., Lippe, B. M. and Gyepes, M. T. (1977). Gray-scale ultrasonography of the normal female pelvis. *Radiology*, **125**, 477–83
21. Orsini, L. F., Salardi, S., Pilu, G., Bovicelli, L. and Cacciari, E. (1984). Pelvic organs in premenarcheal girls: real-time ultrasonography. *Radiology*, **153**, 113–16
22. Ivarsson, S. A., Nilsson, K. O. and Persson, P. H. (1983). Ultrasonography of the pelvic organs in prepubertal and postpubertal girls. *Arch. Dis. Child.*, **58**, 352–4
23. Carlson, B. M. (1981). The development of the urogenital system. In Carlson, B. M. (ed.) *Patten's Foundations of Embryology*, pp. 440–79. (New York: McGraw-Hill)
24. Fritsch, H. (1992). The connective tissue sheath of uterus and vagina in the human female fetus. *Ann. Anat.*, **174**, 261–6
25. Fritsch, H. (1993). Development and organization of the pelvic connective tissue in the human fetus. *Ann. Anat.*, **175**, 531–9
26. Colston Wentz, A. (1988). Congenital anomalies and intersexuality. In Jones III, H. W., Colston Wentz, A. and Burnett, L. S. (eds.) *Novak's Textbook of Gynecology*, pp. 140–86. (Baltimore: Williams & Wilkins)
27. Buttram, V. C. and Gibbons, W. E. (1979). Müllerian anomalies: a proposed classification (an analysis of 144 cases). *Fertil. Steril.*, **32**, 40–6
28. Simón, C., Martinez, L. and Pardo, F. (1991). Müllerian defects in women with normal reproductive outcome. *Fertil. Steril.*, **56**, 1192–3
29. Acién, P. (1993). Reproductive performance of women with uterine malformations. *Hum. Reprod.*, **8**, 122–6
30. Verp, M. S., Simpson, J. L., Elias, S., Carson, S. A., Sarto, G. E. and Feingold, M. (1983). Heritable aspects of uterine anomalies. I Three familial aggregates with Müllerian fusion anomalies. *Fertil. Steril.*, **40**, 80–5
31. Carson, S. A., Simpson, J. L., Malinak, L. R., Elias, S., Gerbie, A. B., Buttram, V. C. and Sarto, G. E. (1983). Heritable aspects of uterine anomalies. II Genetic analysis of Müllerian aplasia. *Fertil. Steril.*, **40**, 86–90
32. Buttram, V. C. (1983). Müllerian anomalies and their management. *Fertil. Steril.*, **40**, 159–63
33. Heinonen, P. K. and Pystynen, P. P. (1983). Primary infertility and uterine anomalies. *Fertil. Steril.*, **40**, 311–16
34. Padykula, H. A. (1988). The female reproductive system. In Weiss, L. (ed.) *Cell and tissue biology*, pp. 866–78 (Baltimore, Munich: Urban & Schwarzenberg)
35. Farrer-Brown, G. and Beilby, J. O. W. (1970). The blood supply of the uterus. I. Arterial vasculature. *J. Obstet. Gynaecol Br. Commonw*, **77**, 673–81
36. Kaisermann-Abramof, I. R. and Padykula, H. A. (1989). Angiogenesis in the preovulatory primate endometrium: the coiled arteriolar system. *Anat. Rec.*, **224**, 479–89
37. Morris, H., Edwards, J., Titman, A. and Emms, M. (1985). Endometrial lymphoid tissue: an immunohistological study. *J. Clin. Pathol.*, **38**, 644–52
38. Staehelin, L. A. (1974). Structure and functions of intercellular junctions. *Int. Ref. Cytol.*, **39**, 191–283
39. Murphy, C. R., Rogers, P. A. W., Hosie, M. J., Leeton, J. and Beaton, L. (1992). Tight junctions of human uterine epithelial cells change during the menstrual cycle: a morphometric study. *Acta Anat.*, **144**, 36–8
40. Murphy, C. R., Swift, J. G., Mukherjee, T. M. and Rogers, A. W. (1982). The structure of tight junctions between uterine luminal epithelial cells at different stages of pregnancy in the rat. *Cell Tissue Res.*, **223**, 281–6
41. Murphy, C. R., Swift, J. G., Need, J. A., Mukherjee, T. M. and Rogers, A. W. (1982). A freeze-fracture electron microscopy study of tight junctions of epithelial cells in the human uterus. *Anat. Embryol.*, **163**, 367–70
42. Rogers, A. W., Murphy, C. R., Leeton, J., Hosie, M. J. and Beaton, L. (1992). Turner's syndrome patients lack tight junction uterine epithelial cells. *Hum. Reprod.*, **7**, 883–5
43. Noyes, R. W., Hertig, A. T. and Rock, J. (1950). Dating the endometrial biopsy. *Fertil. Steril.*, **1**, 3–25
44. Jones III, H. W. (1988). Cyclic histology and cytology of the genital tract. In Jones III, H. W., Wentz, A. C. and Burnett, L. S. (eds.) *Novak's Textbook of Gynecology*, pp. 68–88. (Baltimore: Williams & Wilkins)
45. Wynn, R. M. (1977). Histology and ultrastructure of the human endometrium. In Wynn, R. M. (ed.) *Biology of the Uterus*, pp. 341–76. (New York, London: Plenum Press)
46. Wynn, R. M. and Wooley, R. S. (1967). Ultras-

tructural cyclic changes in the human endometrium. II. Normal postovulatory phase. *Fertil. Steril.*, **18**, 721–38
47. Li, T. C., Rogers, A. W., Lenton, E. A., Dockery, P. and Cooke, I. D. (1987). A comparison between two methods of chronological dating of human endometrial biopsies during the luteal phase and their correlation with histological dating. *Fertil. Steril.*, **48**, 928–33
48. Li, T. C., Rogers, A. W., Dockery, P., Lenton, E. A. and Cooke, I. D. (1988). A new method of histological dating of human endometrium in the luteal phase. *Fertil. Steril.*, **50**, 52–60
49. Dockery, P., Li, T. C., Rogers, A. W., Lenton, E. A., Cooke, I. D. and Warren, M. A. (1988). An examination of the variation in timed endometrial biopsies. *Hum. Reprod.*, **3**, 715–20
50. Dockery, P., Li, T. C., Rogers, A. W., Cooke, I. D. and Lenton, E. A. (1988). The ultrastructure of glandular epithelium in the timed endometrial biopsy. *Hum. Reprod.*, **3**, 826–34
51. Dockery, P., Warren, M. A., Li, T. C., Rogers, A. W. and Cooke, I. D. (1990). A morphometric study of the human endometrial stroma during the peri-implantation period. *Hum. Reprod.*, **5**, 2–9
52. Dockery, P., Tidey, R. R., Li, T. C. and Cooke, I. D. (1991). A morphometric study of the uterine glandular epithelium in women with premature ovarian failure undergoing hormone replacement therapy. *Hum. Reprod.*, **6**, 1354–64
53. Li, T. C., Warren, M. A., Dockery, P. and Cooke, I. D. (1991). Endometrial morphology around the time of implantation in natural and artificial cycles. *J. Reprod. Fertil.*, **92**, (Suppl.), 543–54
54. Li, T., Dockery, P. and Cooke, I. D. (1991). Effects of exogenous progesterone administration on the morphology of normally developing endometrium in the pre-implantation period. *Hum. Reprod.*, **6**, 641–4
55. King, W. J. and Greene, G. L. (1984). Monoclonal antibodies localize oestrogen receptor in the nuclei of target cells. *Nature (London)*, **307**, 745–7
56. Lessey, B. A., Killam, A. P., Metzger, D. A., Haney A. F., Greene, G. L. and McCarty Jr, K. S. (1988). Immunohistochemical analysis of human uterine estrogen and progesterone receptors throughout the menstrual cycle. *J. Clin. Endocrinol. Metab.*, **67**, 334–40
57. Press, M. F., Udove, J. A. and Greene, G. L. (1988). Progesterone receptor distribution in the human endometrium. Analysis using monoclonal antibodies to the human progesterone receptor. *Am. J. Pathol.*, **131**, 112–24
58. Cano, A., Serra, V., Rivera, J., Monmeneu, R. and Marzo, C. (1990). Expression of estrogen receptors, progesterone receptors, and an estrogen receptor-associated protein in the human cervix during the menstrual cycle and menopause. *Fertil. Steril.*, **54**, 1058–64
59. Critchley, H. O. D., Buckley, C. H., Anderson, D. C. and Robertson, W. R. (1992). Expression of an estrogen receptor-related antigen in human endometrium: a microphotometric study. *Hum. Reprod.*, **7**, 151–5
60. Remmele, W., Hildebrand, U., Hienz, A., Klein, P.-J., Vierbuchen, M., Behnken, L. J., Heicke, B. and Scheidt, E. (1986). Comparative histological, histochemical, immunohistochemical and biochemical studies on oestrogen receptors, lecithin receptors, and Barr bodies in human breast cancer. *Virchows Arch. (Pathol. Anat.)*, **409**, 127–47
61. Bur, M. E., Greene, G. L. and Press, M. F. (1987). Estrogen receptor localization in formalin-fixed, paraffin-embedded endometrium and endometriotic tissue. *Int. J. Gynecol Pathol.*, **6**, 140–51
62. Lessey, B. A., Metzger, D. A., Haney, A. F. and McCarty Jr, K. S. (1989). Immuno-histochemical analysis of estrogen and progesterone receptors in endometriosis: comparison with normal endometrium during the menstrual cycle and the effect of medical therapy. *Fertil. Steril.*, **51**, 409–15
63. Lang, G., Lang, M. and Dallenbach-Hellweg, G. (1989). Immuno-histokemische Receptorbefunde in Endometrium und therapeutische Konsequenzen bei endogenen und exogenen Funktionsstörungen und im Karzinom. *Geburtsch. Frauenheilk.*, **49**, 1044–9
64. Bergqvist, A. and Fernö, M. (1993). Estrogen and progesterone receptors in endometriotic tissue and endometrium: comparison according to localization and recurrence. *Fertil. Steril.*, **60**, 63–7
65. Ross, R. and Klebanoff, S. J. (1967). Fine structural changes in uterine smooth muscle and fibroblasts in response to estrogen. *J. Cell Biol.*, **32**, 155–65
66. Haynor, D. R., Mack, L. A., Soules, M. R., Shuman, W. P., Montana, M. A. and Moss, A. A. (1986). Changing appearance of the normal uterus during the menstrual cycle: MR studies. *Radiology*, **161**, 459–62
67. Cullen, B. M. and Harkness, R. D. (1964). Effects of ovariectomy and of hormones on collagenous framework of the uterus. *Am. J. Physiol.*, **206**, 621–7
68. Fainstat, T. (1962). Hormonal basis for collagen bundle generation in uterine stroma: extracellular studies of uterus. *Endocrinology*, **71**, 878–92
69. Woessner Jr, J. F. and Brewer, T. H. (1963). Formation and breakdown of collagen and elastin in the human uterus during pregnancy and postpartum involution. *Biochem. J.*, **89**, 75–9
70. Laguens, R. and Lagrutta, J. (1964). Fine structure of human uterine muscle in pregnancy. *Am. J. Obstet. Gynecol.*, **89**, 1040–7
71. Fawcett, D. W. (1986). Muscular tissue. In Fawcett, D. W. (ed.) *A Textbook of Histology*, pp. 265–310. (Philadelphia, London, Toronto: W. B. Saunders)
72. Decker, R. S. (1976). Hormonal regulation of gap junction differentiation. *J. Cell Biol.*, **69**, 669–85

73. Fuchs, A. R. (1977). Prostaglandins. In Fuchs, F. and Klopper, A. (eds.) *Endocrinology of Pregnancy*, pp. 294–326. (New York: Harper and Row)
74. Garfield, R. E., Sims, S. and Daniel, E. E. (1977). Gap junctions: their presence and necessity in myometrium during parturition. *Science*, **198**, 958–60
75. Garfield, R. E., Sims, S. M., Kannan, M. S. and Daniel, E. E. (1978). The possible role of gap junctions in activation of the myometrium during parturition. *Am. J. Physiol.*, **235**, C168–79
76. Garfield, R. E., Kannan, M. S. and Daniel, E. E. (1980). Gap junction formation in myometrium: control by estrogens, progesterone, and prostaglandins. *Am. J. Physiol.*, **238**, C81–9
77. Garfield, R. E., Merrett, D. and Grover, A. K. (1980). Gap junction formation and regulation in myometrium. *Am. J. Physiol.*, **239**, C217–28
78. Scoutt, L. M., McCarthy, S. M., Flynn, S. D., Luthringer, D. J. and McCarthy, S. M. (1993). Zonal anatomy of the cervix: correlation of MR imaging and histologic examination of hysterectomy specimens. *Radiology*, **186**, 159–62

Uterine perfusion

10

S. Kupesic and A. Kurjak

INTRODUCTION

More than any other available technique, transvaginal color Doppler affords detailed delineation of the uterus, its myometrium, endometrium and vessels[1].

The vascular supply to the uterus is provided by a complex network of arteries originating from the uterine artery, which is a branch of the hypogastric artery. The color Doppler signal from the main uterine vessels can be seen lateral to the cervix at the level of the cervicocorporeal junction of the uterus[2]. Its main branches extend inward for about a third of the myometrium, forming the arcuate wreath which encircles the uterus[3]. Smaller branches, called radial arteries, are directed towards the uterine lumen[4]. When passing the inner third of the myometrium and myometrioendometrial junction, they become spiral arteries.

It is well known that uterine perfusion is largely dependent on the patient's age, phase of the menstrual cycle, and other specific conditions (e.g. pregnancy, tumor)[5]. In this chapter, we analyze them in detail.

UTERINE PERFUSION CHANGES DURING THE MENSTRUAL CYCLE

There are complex relationships between the concentration of the ovarian hormones in peripheral venous plasma and uterine artery blood flow parameters[6–9]. In most women, there is a small amount of end-diastolic flow in the uterine arteries in the proliferative phase (Figure 1). The resistance index hovers around 0.88 ± 0.04 until day 13 of the 28-day menstrual cycle (Color plate D). Steer and co-workers[8] reported that diastolic flow in the uterine arteries disappeared during the day of ovulation. Goswamy and Steptoe[6] found increasing resistance index and systolic/diastolic ratio during the postovulatory drop in the serum estradiol concentration. Increased uterine artery impedance was reported 3 days after the peak in luteinizing hormone (LH), and Scholtes and colleagues[10] recorded the highest value for the pulsatility index (PI) in the uterine arteries on cycle day 16.

These findings may be explained by increased uterine contractility[11] and compression of the vessels traversing the uterine wall, which decrease their diameter and consequently cause higher resistance to flow. During the normal menstrual cycle, there is a sharp increase in end-diastolic velocities between the proliferative and secretory phases[2]. It is particularly interesting that the lowest blood flow impedance occurs during the time of peak luteal function (resistance index (RI) $= 0.84 \pm 0.04$), during which implantation is most likely to occur (Color plate E). It is logical that blood supply to the uterus should be high in the late luteal phase, as has been reported by Kurjak and associates[2], Goswamy and associates[6,7], Steer and associates[8], and Battaglia and associates[12]. The persistently lower RI in the luteal phase suggests that the relaxation effects on the uterine arteries persist until the onset of menstruation.

Similar circulatory changes to those observed in the main uterine arteries have been seen in the minute arteries (radial and spiral) with the introduction of transvaginal color and pulsed Doppler[13]. Our results show an increase of the RI in the myometrial vessels after ovulation, during the postovulatory drop in the serum estradiol concentration (Color plate F).

Increased uterine contractility has been shown to coincide with decreased endometrial blood flow[11]. It is well known that the endometrium has an exceptional capacity to undergo changes in

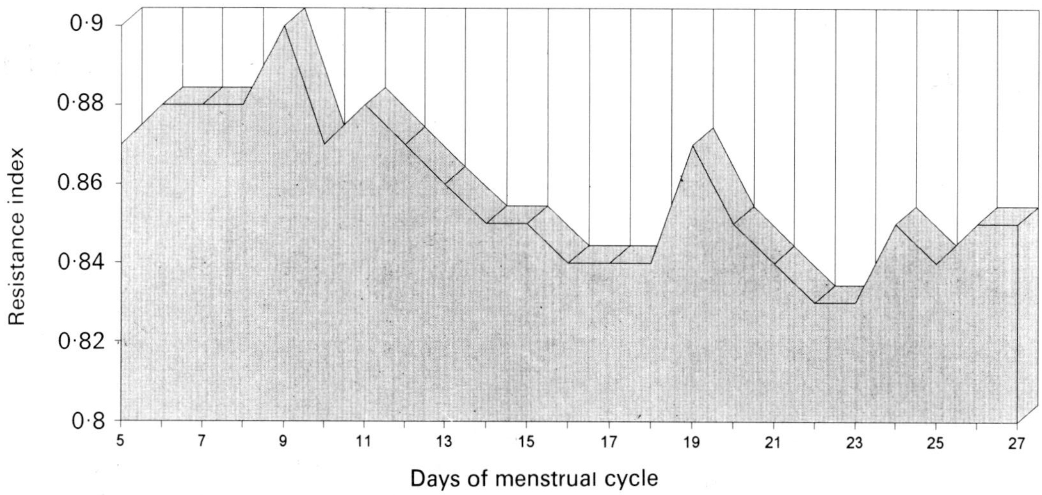

Figure 1 Uterine artery flow velocity during the menstrual cycle in ovulatory women ($n=72$)

structure and function during the menstrual cycle. The histological changes include striking development of the blood vessels. The spiral arteries become more developed during the menstrual cycle. The increased endometrial vascularity is highly dependent upon the uterine, arcuate and radial artery blood flow. Blood flow velocity waveform changes in the spiral arteries during normal ovulatory cycles are characterized by lower velocity ($p<0.05$) and lower impedance to blood flow ($p<0.05$) than are those observed in the uterine arteries, with larger diameter[14] (Color plate G). It seems that features of endometrial blood flow may be used to predict the implantation success rate and to reveal unexplained infertility problems more precisely than evaluation of the main uterine artery alone.

UTERINE PERFUSION IN INFERTILE PATIENTS

The expanding experience with transvaginal color and pulsed Doppler sonography has established this technique as an additional tool in the management of infertile patients. In anovulatory cycles, a continuous increase of the uterine artery RI has been detected[2]. Moreover, in some infertile patients, and end-diastolic flow is absent[7] (Color plate H). There are not enough data to speculate whether absent diastolic flow is associated with infertility and poor reproductive performance.

The uterine artery blood flow could be used to predict a hostile uterine environment prior to embryo transfer[8]. It is possible to calculate the probability of pregnancy by using PI values obtained from the uterine artery on the day of embryo transfer. With the use of these measurements, the highest probability of becoming pregnant was obtained in those patients with medium values of uterine artery PI[8]. A mean PI of more than 3.0 before the transfer can predict up to 35% of failures to become pregnant. However, more studies are necessary to establish the precise relationship between uterine artery perfusion and the probability of pregnancy. Those women with poor uterine perfusion could be advised to have their embryos cryopreserved for transfer at a later date.

An improvement of the uterine blood flow may be achieved by administration of estradiol[15] and perhaps even progesterone[16]. One of the major problems associated with current practice in *in vitro* fertilization is the necessity to use multiple embryo transfer to increase the pregnancy rate. This leads to an increased incidence of multiple pregnancy. This may contribute to increased obstetric risk and poorer perinatal outcome, when compared to singleton pregnancies. It is well known that the probability of pregnancy is strongly related to embryo quality and uterine receptivity. Instead of by endometrial biopsy, which may cause trauma and bleeding at the

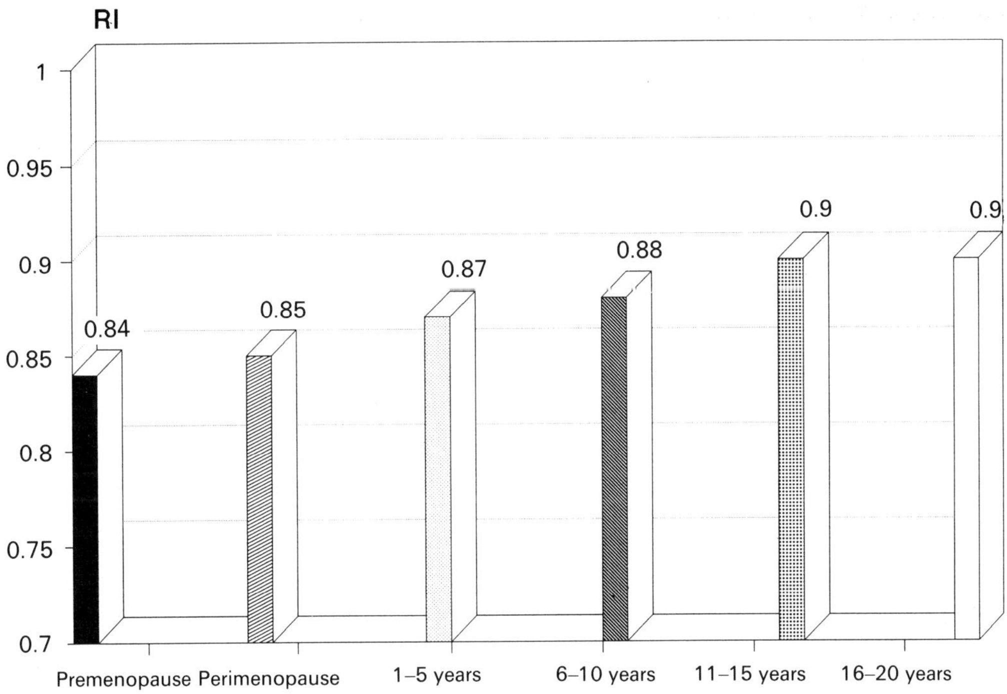

Figure 2 Uterine artery resistance index in women of premenopausal age ($n=22$), perimenopausal age ($n=28$) and postmenopausal age ($n=85$)

implantation site, uterine receptivity should be assessed by color Doppler ultrasound. This easily repeatable procedure is rapid, simple to perform and may predict the likelihood of implantation, minimizing the risk of multiple pregnancy. Studies of uterine blood flow might become a non-invasive assay of uterine receptivity, giving us more information on the pathophysiology of infertility, especially in the group of patients with unexplained causes.

UTERINE BLOOD FLOW IN POSTMENOPAUSAL WOMEN

The ageing process and its influence on the endometrium, myometrium and total size of the uterus has been previously studied[17,18]. It is reported that endometrial and myometrial thickness are changed as the years of the postmenopause progress. Myometrial thickness after the menopause changes less than does endometrial thickness, which may suggest that these changes are more dynamic.

Our recent study[19] included 85 healthy postmenopausal women examined by transvaginal color Doppler. Patients with uterine and adnexal abnormalities, as well as those receiving hormonal replacement therapy, were excluded from the study. They were divided into subgroups according to the duration of the postmenopause (1–5 years, 6–10 years, 11–15 years and over 16 years). Uterine morphology and perfusion were assessed in all patients. Visualization of both uterine arteries was achieved in all women, while radial arteries were identified in 71.8%. The visualization rate of the myometrial and endometrial vessels was highly dependent on the length of the postmenopausal period. Low visualization of the endometrial vessels was in accordance with the fact that mean thickness of the endometrium was 0.7 cm in the group of patients with 1–5 years of postmenopause, 0.5 cm in the group with 6–10 years of postmenopause, and 0.4 cm in the group with more than 11 years of postmenopause. The resistance to blood flow in the uterine arteries is shown in Figure 2.

The ageing process affects uterine perfusion. Resistance to blood flow increases in both the main uterine and the radial arteries as the years of postmenopause progress. The effect of the gonadal hormones and hormonal replacement therapy on the uterine arterial tone is discussed elsewhere in this book.

References

1. Kurjak, A. and Kupesic-Urek, S. (1992). Normal and abnormal uterine perfusion. In Jaffe, R. and Warsof, L. S. (eds.) *Color Doppler Imaging in Obstetrics and Gynecology*, pp. 255–63. (New York: McGraw Hill)
2. Kurjak, A., Kupesic-Urek, S., Schulman, H. and Zalud, I. (1991). Transvaginal color flow Doppler in the assessment of ovarian and uterine blood flow in infertile women. *Fertil. Steril.*, **56**, 870–3
3. Du Bose, T. J., Hill, L. W. and Henningan, J. W. Jr (1985). Sonography of arcuate uterine blood vessels. *J. Ultrasound Med.*, **4**, 229–33
4. Jurkovic, D., Jauniaux, E., Kurjak, A. and Campbell, S. (1991). Transvaginal color Doppler assessment of the uteroplacental circulation in early pregnancy. *Obstet. Gynecol.*, **77**, 365–9
5. Long, M. G., Boultbee, J. E., Hanson, M. E. and Begent, J. H. R. (1989). Doppler time velocity waveform studies of the uterine artery and uterus. *Br. J. Obstet. Gynaecol.*, **96**, 588–93
6. Goswamy, R. K. and Steptoe, P. C. (1988). Doppler ultrasound studies of the uterine artery in spontaneous ovarian cycles. *Hum. Reprod.*, **3**, 721–3
7. Goswamy, R. K., Williams, G. and Steptoe, P. C. (1988). Decreased uterine perfusion a cause of infertility. *Hum. Reprod.*, **3**, 955–8
8. Steer, C. V., Mills, C. V. and Campbell, S. (1991). Vaginal color Doppler assessment on the day of embryo transfer (ET) accurately predicts patients in an *in vitro* fertilization programme with suboptimal uterine perfusion who fail to become pregnant. *Ultrasound. Obstet. Gynecol.*, **1**, 79–82
9. Bourne, T. H., Jurkovic, D., Waterstone, J., Campbell, S. and Collins, W. P. (1991). Intrafollicular blood flow during human ovulation. *Ultrasound Obstet. Gynecol.*, **1**, 53–7
10. Scholtes, M. C. W., Wladimiroff, J. W., van Rijen, H. J. M. and Hop, W. C. J. (1989). Uterine and ovarian flow velocity waveforms in the normal menstrual cycle: a transvaginal study. *Fertil. Steril.*, **52**, 981–5
11. Hauksson, A., Akerlund, M. and Melin, P. (1988). Uterine blood flow and myometrial activity at menstruation, and the action of vasopressin and a synthetic antagonist. *Br. J. Obstet. Gynaecol.*, **95**, 898–904
12. Battaglia, C., Larocca, E., Lanzani, A., Valentini, M. and Genanzzani, A. R. (1990). Doppler ultrasound studies of the uterine arteries in spontaneous and IVF cycles. *Gynecol. Endocrinol.*, **4**, 245–50
13. Kupesic, S. and Kurjak, A. (1993). Uterine and ovarian perfusion during the periovulatory period assessed by transvaginal color Doppler. *Fertil. Steril.*, **60**, 439–43
14. Kupesic, S., Kurjak, A. and Stilinovic, K. (1994). The assessment of female infertility. In Kurjak, A. (ed.) *An Atlas of Transvaginal Color Doppler*, pp. 171–99. (Carnforth, UK: Parthenon Publishing)
15. Ford, S. P., Reynolds, R. P. and Farley, D. B. (1984). Interaction of ovarian steroids and periarterial alpha-1-adrenergic receptors in altering uterine blood flow during the estrous cycle of gilts. *Am. J. Obstet. Gynecol.*, **150**, 480–4
16. de Ziegler, D., Bessis, R. and Frydman, R. (1991). Vascular resistance of uterine arteries: physiological effects of estradiol and progesterone. *Fertil. Steril.*, **55**, 775–8
17. Varner, R. E., Sparks, J. M. and Cameron, C. D. (1991). Transvaginal sonography of the endometrium in postmenopausal women. *Obstet. Gynecol.*, **78**, 195–200
18. Zalud, I., Conway, C., Schulman, H. and Trinc, D. (1993). Endometrial and myometrial thickness and uterine blood flow in postmenopausal women. *J. Ultrasound Med.*, **12**, 737–41
19. Kurjak, A. and Kupesic, S. (1994). Aging in women: the significance of uterine and ovarian perfusion. *Fertil. Steril.*, submitted

Drug influence on uterine perfusion 11

S. Kupesic and A. Kurjak

EFFECT OF ESTRADIOL AND PROGESTERONE ON VASCULAR RESISTANCE

Rhythmic changes in uterine blood flow during the estrous cycle in different species are temporally associated with the daily ratio of estrogen to progesterone in systemic blood[1–3]. The higher the estrogen : progesterone ratio, the greater the quantity of blood flow through the uterine vascular bed[4–6]. Progesterone antagonizes the uterine vasodilatory effect of estrogen[7,8], and the magnitude of this inhibition is related to the ratio of the two steroids[7].

The uterine periarterial symphathetic vasoconstrictor nerves have been postulated as being important in regulating uterine blood flow[9]. Exposure to progesterone has been shown to increase, whereas estrogen decreases, the function of uterine periarterial symphathetic vasoconstrictor nerves[10,11]. The results of Ford and colleagues[12] suggest that ovarian steroids alter the function of uterine periarterial sympathetic nerves through changes in α-adrenergic receptor numbers, which may contribute to the marked changes in uterine blood flow observed during the porcine estrous cycle.

To clarify the role played by physiological levels of ovarian hormones in the vascular resistance of uterine arteries, De Ziegler and associates[13] conducted a study in young women deprived of ovarian function who received physiological estradiol and progesterone replacement therapy. Their results showed that in the absence of estrogen production by the ovary, uterine arteries have a high degree of vascular resistance, expressed by narrow systolic Doppler flow waves and high values of the pulsatility index (PI).

According to the hypothesis of Goswamy and Steptoe[14], multiparous women have persistent diastolic flow during the early follicular phase more often than do nulliparous women. A profound modification of the Doppler flow pattern, suggesting a marked decrease in vascular resistance, was detected after the transdermal administration of estradiol (0.1–0.4 mg/day). This observation is in accordance with the hypothesis that the decrease in vascular resistance observed at the time of ovulation is mediated by estradiol[15]. Because estrogen receptors have been identified in the walls of the uterine arteries, it is likely that the effect of estradiol on the uterine waveform is direct. Therefore, it is postulated that the estrogenic effect on the uterine artery vascular resistance is directly related to the plasma level of biologically active estrogens and that a direct dose–effect relationship exists[16].

Other possible mechanisms include modulation by estradiol of the production and/or secretion of certain vasoactive substances, such as prostaglandins[17], calcitonin gene-related peptide[18] and endothelial relaxing factor[19]. Undoubtedly, transvaginal Doppler studies of the uterine arteries are a valuable reflector of the biological efficacy of various estrogenic treatments. This is particularly important for evaluating the effects of the postmenopausal hormonal replacement regimens in women who have an increased hepatic metabolism of estrogen and, therefore, lower levels of plasma estradiol.

The influence of progesterone on the PI in humans has not yet been determined. In lower mammals, progesterone acts as a vasoconstrictor[20,21]. This raises the concern that the progesterone that is added in estrogen replacement therapy, either sequentially or continuously, for endometrial protection[21] may partially or totally reverse the apparent vasodilatory action of estrogen. Hillard and associates[21] used transvaginal color and pulsed Doppler to measure the PI in the uterine arteries before and during the estradiol and estradiol/progesterone treatment. In all patients, the addition of norethindrone acetate (0.7 mg/day) or medroxyprogesterone acetate (10 mg/day) partially antagonized the response to transdermal estradiol. The PI was approximately 34% lower than the pretreatment value during the combined estradiol/progestrone phase of treatment, but 13% higher when compared with the estradiol only treatment phase. It remains unclear whether the effects of the progesterone on the uterine artery PI are correlated with the clinical reduction in arterial disease protection with estrogen replacement therapy.

The next step will be to determine whether a reduction in uterine artery impedance correlates with arterial disease protection. Furthermore, a threshold value, below which a further reduction in the PI or resistance index (RI) is not associated with greater protection from arterial disease, should be estimated.

Goswamy and Steptoe[14] have assessed uterine perfusion in a population of infertile patients who failed to achieve pregnancy after three previous completed treatment cycles for *in vitro* fertilization (IVF). Of these patients, 48% were noted to have abnormal uterine perfusion. Possible explanations for the decreased uterine perfusion response are decreased uterine receptivity to endogenous hormones, or the decreased sensitivity of the uterus due to the desensitization effect of endogenous hormones. Most of the patients (86%) improved their response on high doses of estradiol–valerate therapy. The pregnancy rate achieved after improving uterine perfusion was comparable to or even better than that obtained in the control group.

EFFECT OF GnRH ANALOGS ON UTERINE BLOOD FLOW

The postmenopause is a phase of life in which genital organs undergo numerous changes, mostly induced by low levels of estrogens. In the spontaneous menopause, disappearance of the follicular units and reduction of estrogen secretion are followed by an increase in hypophyseal gonadotropin secretion. The uterus shows an atrophic endometrium and an increase in the number of stromal cells within the myometrium. Diminished thickness of the vaginal and vulvar mucosa and increased vaginal dryness are features[22].

Menopausal women show increased whole blood viscosity, plasma viscosity and red cell rigidity[23]. All these changes are attributable to the significant changes in blood rheology. The complex relationship between the concentration of female hormones in peripheral venous plasma and uterine artery blood flow were successfully demonstrated by Doppler studies[24,25]. The uterine artery blood flow is diminished in the menopause and the impedance to blood flow in uterine arteries increases with the years from the cessation of menses[26].

The induction of an artificial menopause with analogs of gonadotropin releasing hormone (GnRH) has shown good biological tolerability, while the mechanism of their linkage with hypophyseal receptors causes temporary and reversible diminution of their number and causes the suppression of gonadotropin levels and hypostimulation of the ovaries[27].

In this chapter, we evaluate uterine perfusion by means of color Doppler velocimetry in four groups of patients: fertile healthy volunteers in late luteal phase, those with uterine fibroids who received GnRH analogs for 6 months, climacteric women after at least 5 years of menopause and infertile patients undergoing IVF after long pretreatment with GnRH analogs.

UTERINE PERFUSION IN DIFFERENT GROUPS

The subjects of our study (S. Kupesic and A. Kurjak, unpublished data) were 165 patients: 50 healthy and normally menstruating women, 25 patients with uterine fibroids who had undergone pharmacological treatment with GnRH analogs for under 6 months, 50 women at least 5 years after spontaneous menopause and 40 IVF patients after long pretreatment with GnRH analogs. The flow velocity waveform of the main branch of the uterine artery was detected lateral to the supravaginal portion of the cervix, and the mean RI was calculated. In the group composed of normally menstruating healthy volunteers, the flow velocity waveform study of the uterine arteries was

Table 1 Doppler studies of uterine arteries in healthy volunteers, women with artificially induced menopause and uterine fibroids (uterine fibroids), menopausal women with uterine fibroids (menopausal patients), and menopausal patients and candidates for *in vitro* fertilization after long pretreatment with GnRH analogs (GnRH analogs)

	Controls	*Uterine fibroids*	*Menopausal patients*	*GnRH analogs*
Number				
Age (years)	50	25	50	40
mean	37	39	50	33
range	28–42	31–47	51–61	28–42
Uterine artery mean RI (±SD)	0.84±0.08	before: 0.74±0.07 after: 0.88±0.04	0.91±0.04	0.80±0.04

performed in the mid-luteal phase (21st day of the menstrual cycle). The mean age of the patients was 37 years (range 28–42 years). In the group of patients with uterine fibroids, the first examination was performed in the mid-luteal phase, before the start of GnRH analog treatment, and the second examination was performed after 6 months of the treatment. The mean age in this group was 39 years (range 31–47 years). The third group consisted of postmenopausal women (more than 5 years after cessation of menses). Their mean age was 58 years (range 51–61 years). In the fourth group (IVF patients after long inhibition with GnRH analogs) the uterine artery blood flow analysis was performed the day after oocyte aspiration. The mean age in this group was 33 years (range 28–42 years).

For all groups, the mean and standard deviation of the uterine artery RI were calculated. The differences were analyzed by means of the one-way analysis of variance (ANOVA) test. A value of $p<0.05$ was considered statistically significant. Results are shown in Table 1.

In the healthy fertile volunteers, the mid-luteal RI of the uterine arteries was 0.84±0.08. The mean RI of the uterine arteries in patients with uterine fibroids during the mid-luteal phase before GnRH analog treatment was 0.74±0.07. After 6 months' treatment, the mean RI was significantly increased, with the value of 0.88±0.04. In the group of postmenopausal patients, the mean RI was 0.91.±0.04. In the group of IVF patients after long pretreatment with GnRH analogs, the uterine artery RI the day after oocyte aspiration (the day before expected embryo transfer) was 0.82±0.008.

A statistically significant difference was detected in the mean uterine artery RI in the mid-luteal phase between the first and second groups, and in the mean RI in menopause, between the group treated with GnRH analogs and the group with spontaneous menopause. There was no statistically significant difference between the uterine artery RI of the healthy controls in mid-luteal phase and the IVF patients.

It is well known that uterine perfusion depends on female hormone variations and that the lowest flow impedance occurs during the time of peak luteal function[24]. Our study demonstrates diminished uterine artery perfusion in postmenopausal patients. Diastolic flow decreases in the menopause, showing a progressively deepening notch or even totally absent diastolic flow. Patients with artificially induced menopause show higher vascular compliance, demonstrated by high diastolic flow and a shallower notch. This difference may be due to a different hormonal milieu, because gonadotropins induce the secretion of both vasodilators (prostaglandin E_2; PGE_2) and vasoconstrictors (PGF_{2a}). Furthermore, the increased uterine artery RI should be related to the level of hypergonadotropinemia, progressive sclerosis of the vessel wall and hemorrheological changes.

Uterine perfusion in patients with uterine leiomyoma after 6 months' GnRH analog treatment

Uterine leiomyomas are the most common solid pelvic tumors, typical of the reproductive age, which tend to regress spontaneously after the menopause[28]. Leiomyomas contain more high-affinity estrogen receptors than does neighbouring uterine muscle. To induce their growth or to maintain their size, they depend upon estrogen via a direct or indirect mechanism[29]. Treatment with gonadotropin releasing hormone agonists (GnRHa) induces a reversible state of hypogonadism and is reported to have a positive effect on leiomyomas[30].

Twenty-five patients with uterine fibroids were included in the study. All had symptoms: metrorrhagia (88%), pelvic discomfort and/or pain (52%) and dysmenorrhea (40%). Each patient underwent transabdominal and/or transvaginal sonography, during which the uterus and both adnexa were examined. The fibroid volume was calculated with the formula for an ellipsoid (0.521 × length × width × depth). Color and pulsed Doppler were used for identification and quantification of the blood flow of the main arteries supplying the uterine tumor. Introductory discussions were held on uterine artery perfusion with this group of patients. The initial fibroid volume ranged from 25 to 390 mm^3 (mean 85 mm^3). Buserelin (Suprefact, Hoechst) was given 1200 μg/day intranasally. Follow-up consisted of transvaginal color Doppler examination during, and at the end of, the GnRH analog treatment.

The mean RI measured in the main arteries supplying the tumor was 0.54 ± 0.08. The impedance in these vessels increased sharply during the first 3 months of treatment (mean RI = 0.78), while the mean fibroid volume decreased to 76% of the initial size. After 6 months' therapy, fibroid size was reduced to 56% of the initial volume, while in 80% of patients, color Doppler showed further reduction in the main uterine artery (mean RI = 0.88) and major fibroid arteries (mean RI = 0.82) (Figure 1).

Furthermore, three fibroids had regressed completely and did not grow in the 6-month period after the end of the treatment. The rest had increased their volume to 24% of the post-treatment value. Nine patients were brought to the surgery, with increased hemoglobin concentration, reduced uterine and fibroid volume – which allowed surgery (myomectomy or hysterectomy) – reduced intraoperative bleeding – allowing easier removal of the myomatous tissue – and decreased rate of postoperative complications[30,31]. Furthermore, four perimenopausal patients with severe metrorrhagia passed to complete menopause.

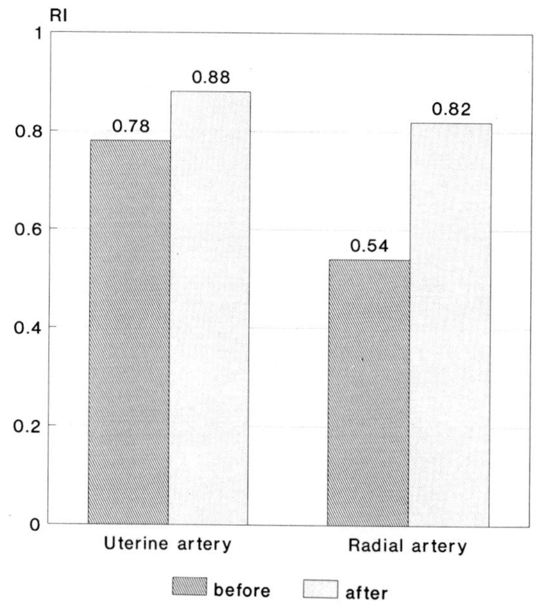

Figure 1 Resistance index (RI) of the uterine and radial arteries in patients with fibroids, before and after 6 months of treatment with gonadotropin releasing hormone analogs

Uterine perfusion in IVF patients with long GnRH pretreatment

Effective superovulation is essential for *in vitro* fertilization, as rates of pregnancy are related to the number of good-quality oocytes recovered and fertilized and the number of embryos transferred to the uterus. GnRH analogs abolish the spontaneous release of gonadotropins by the pituitary gland and protect oocytes from inappropriate exposure to LH, which is thought to be detrimental to normal maturation of the egg[27]. Such a temporary hypogonadotropic hypogonadism allows follicles to be stimulated by exogeneous human menopausal gonadotropin (hMG) or follicle stimulating hormone (FSH) earlier in the follicular recruitment process.

Our study group consisted of 40 patients who were receiving 'long' GnRH pretreatment. Buserelin was given at a dose of 1200 μg per day intranasally. Exogenous gonadotropins (hMG) were started when the LH provocation test was negative. The uterine artery RI the day after oocyte aspiration was lower (mean RI =

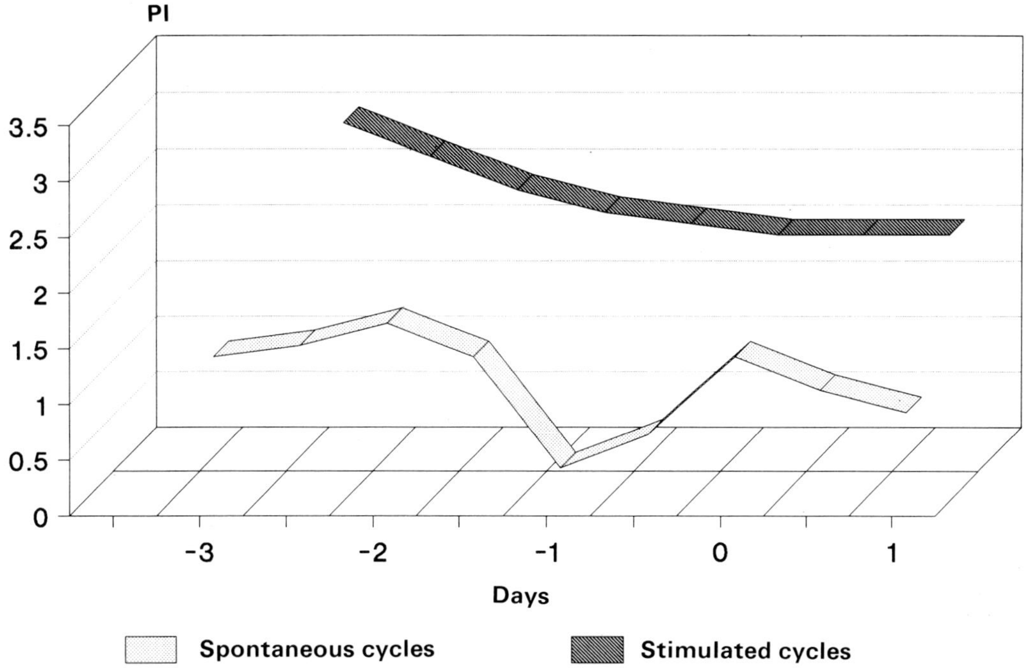

Figure 2 Uterine artery blood flow in spontaneous and stimulated cycles

0.80 ⊥ 0.04) than observed in the mid-luteal phase of the healthy fertile controls.

In the study of Linder and associates[2] pregnancy per transfer rate was 25%, compared with 11% in the hMG-treated group. Rutherford and co-workers[33] demonstrated that the mean number of oocytes recovered was significantly higher (9.5 vs. 5.5), as was the mean number of embryos obtained (4.3 vs. 2.9) with GnRH analog therapy. Undoubtedly, this treatment allowed a better follicular response and higher implantation rate, due to the implantation of more embryos and to their appropriate selection. It is hoped that a prospective longitudinal study with transvaginal color Doppler will include more patients, and confirm the increased uterine perfusion and receptivity, with the use of this treatment protocol.

Uterine perfusion in spontaneous and induced ovarian cycles with confirmed ovulation

Kupesic and Kurjak[34] measured the flow velocity of the uterine, radial and spiral arteries during the periovulatory period in spontaneous and induced ovarian cycles with confirmed ovulation. They studied daily measurements of 78 patients attending an infertility clinic, because of the male factor in infertility.

In spontaneous cycles, the uterine flow velocity had a PI of 3.16, 2 days before ovulation, and started to decrease the day before ovulation (PI = 2.22). In stimulated cycles, these changes did not occur, and the mean PI of 3.06 remained at that level during the periovulatory period (Figure 2). Clear flow velocity waveforms were obtained from the endometrium and myometrium at around the time of ovulation. The pulsatility indices of radial and spiral arteries showed significantly higher values in stimulated than in spontaneous cycles.

Clomiphene citrate is known to deplete estrogen receptors in estrogen-sensitive tissues, influencing endometrial growth and pattern[35]. There was a strong correlation between endometrial thickness and flow velocities. However, this did not apply to the group of patients stimulated with clomiphene citrate/hMG and normal endometrial growth, where the authors demonstrated the absence of diastolic flow in spiral arteries in 55.6% of patients. However, no difference in endometrial thickness and perfusion was observed between hMG-stimulated patients and those in spontaneous cycles. Indeed. spiral artery blood flow changes may be used as an accurate predictor of implantation success rate in treatment with IVF/embryo transfer. Those women with poor uterine perfusion in their current treatment cycles could be advised to have their embryos cryopreserved and transferred either in a spontaneous cycle or after correction of the endometrial perfusion by an appropriate treatment (e.g. estradiol valerate).

References

1. Ford, S. P., Chenault, J. R. and Echterncamp S. E. (1979). Uterine blood flow of cows during the estrous cycle and early pregnancy: effect of the conceptus on the uterine blood supply. *J. Reprod. Fertil.*, **56**, 53–8
2. Yuthasastrakosol, P., Palmer, W.M. and Howland, B. E. (1975). Luteinizing hormone, oestrogen and progesterone levels in peripheral serum of anoestrous and cyclic ewes as determined by radioimmunoassay. *J. Reprod. Fertil.*, **43**, 57–62
3. Henricks, D. M., Guthlie, H. D. and Handlin, D. L. (1975). Plasma estrogen, progesterone and luteinizing hormone levels during the estrous cycle in pigs. *Biol. Reprod.*, **6**, 210–16
4. Killam, A. P., Rosenfeld C., Battaglia, F. C., Makowski, E. L. and Meschia, G. (1973). Effect of estrogens on the uterine blood flow in oophorectemized ewes. *Am. J. Obstet. Gynecol.*, **115**, 1045–50
5. Ford, S. P. and Reynolds, L. P. (1983). Role of adrenergic receptors in mediating estradiol-17 beta stimulated increases in uterine blood flow of cows. *J. Anim. Sci.*, **57**, 665–9
6. Dickson, W. M., Bosc, M. J. and Locatelli, A. (1969). Effect of estrogen and progesterone on uterine blood flow in castrate sows. *Am. J. Physiol.*, **217**, 1431–7
7. Caton, D., Abrams, R. M., Clapp, J. F. and Barron, D. (1974). The effect of exogenous progesterone on the rate of blood flow of the uterus of ovariectomized sheep. *Q. J. Exp. Physiol.*, **59**, 225–31
8. Resnik, R., Brink, G. W. and Plumer, M. H. (1977). The effect of progestrone on estrogen-induced uterine blood flow. *Am. J. Obstet. Gynecol.*, **128**, 251–5
9. Ford, S. P. (1973). Control of uterine and ovarian blood flow throughout the estrous cycle and pregnancy of the ewe, sow and cow. *J. Anim. Sci.*, **55** (Suppl. 2), 32–4
10. Ford, S. P., Weber, L. J. and Stormshak, F. (1976). *In vitro* response of ovine and bovine uterine arteries to prostaglandin $F_{2\alpha}$ and periarterial sympathetic nerve stimulation. *Biol. Reprod.*, **15**, 58–64
11. Ford, S. P., Weber, L. J. and Stormshak, F. (1977). Role of estradiol 17 beta and progesterone in regulating constriction of ovine arteries. *Biol. Reprod.*, **17**, 480–6
12. Ford, S. P., Reynolds, L. P., Farley, D. B., Bhatnagar, R. K. and van Orden, D. E. (1984). Interaction of ovarian steroids and periarterial alpha-1-adrenergic receptors in altering uterine blood flow during the estrous cycle of gilts. *Am. J. Obstet. Gynecol.*, **5**, 480–4
13. De Ziegler, D., Bessis, R. and Frydman, R. (1991). Vascular resistance of uterine arteries: physiological effects of estradiol and progesterone. *Fertil. Steril.*, **55**, 775–9
14. Goswamy, R. K. and Steptoe, P. C. (1988). Doppler ultrasound studies of the uterine artery in spontaneous ovarian cycles. *Hum. Reprod.*, **3**, 721–5
15. Perrot-Applanat, M., Groyer-Picart, M. T., Garcia, E., Lorenzo, F. and Milgrom, E. (1988). Immunocytochemical demonstration of estrogen and progesterone receptors in muscle cells of uterine arteries in rabbits and humans. *Endocrinology*, **123**, 1511–14
16. Sarrel, P. M. (1990). Ovarian hormones and circulation. *Maturitas*, **590**, 297–8
17. Steinleitner, A., Stancyzk, F. Z., Levin, J. N., d'Ablaing, G., Vijod, M. A. and Shabhagian, V. L. (1989). Decreased *in vitro* production of 6-keto-prostaglandin $F_{1\alpha}$ by uterine arteries from postmenopausal women. *Am. J. Obstet. Gynecol.*, **161**, 1677–81
18. Stevenson, J. C., McDonald, D. W. R., Waren, R. C., Booker, M. W. and Whitehead, M. I. (1986). Increased concentration of circulating calcitonin gene related peptide during normal human pregnancy. *Br. Med. J.*, **29**, 1329–30
19. Furchgott, R. F. and Zawadzki, J. W. (1980). The obligatory role of endothelial cells in the relaxation of arterial smooth muscle by acetyl choline. *Nature (London)*, **288**, 373–6
20. Resnik, R. (1976). The effect of progesterone on estrogen induced uterine blood flow. *Gynecol. Invest.*, **128**, 251–4

21. Hillard, T. C., Bourne, T., Whitehead, M. I., Cryford, T. B., Collins W. P. and Campbell, S. (1992). Differential effects of transdermal estradiol and sequential progestogens on impedance to flow within the uterine arteries of postmenopausal women. *Fertil. Steril.*, **58**, 959–63
22. London, S. N. and Hammond, C. B. (1990). The climacteric. In Scott, J. R., DiSaia, P. J., Hammond, C. B. and Spellacy, W. N. (eds.) *Danforth's Obstetrics and Gynecology*, pp. 853–73. (Philadelphia: JB Lippincott)
23. Puniyami, R. R. and Sonar, S. (1991). Hemorrheological changes at menopause. *Clin. Hemorrheol.*, **11**, 397–402
24. Kurjak, A., Kupesic-Urek, S., Schulman, H. and Zalud, I. (1991). Transvaginal color Doppler in the assessment of ovarian and uterine perfusion in infertile women. *Fertil. Steril.*, **6**, 870–4
25. Steer, C. V., Campbell, S., Pampiglione, J., Kingsland, C., Mason, B. A. and Collins, W. P. (1990). Transvaginal color flow imaging of uterine arteries during the ovarian and menstrual cycle. *Hum. Reprod.*, **5**, 391–5
26. Kurjak, A., Shalan, H., Kupesic, S., Predanic, M., Zalud, I., Breyer, B. and Jukic, S. (1993). Transvaginal color Doppler sonography in the assessment of pelvic tumor vascularity. *Ultrasound Obstet. Gynecol.*, **3**, 1–18
27. Karten, M. J. and River, J. (1986). Gonadotropin-releasing hormone analogue design structure–function studies toward the development of agonist and antagonist. Rationale and perspectives. *Endocr. Rev.*, **7**, 44–56
28. Lumesden, M. A., West, C. P. and Baird, D. T. (1987). Goserelin therapy before surgery for uterine fibroids. *Lancet*, **1**, 33–4
29. Buttram, V. C. and Reiter, R. C. (1981). Uterine leiomyomata: etiology, syptomatology and management. *Fertil. Steril.*, **36**, 433–5
30. Maheux, R., Guilloteau, C., Lemay, A., Bastide, A. and Fazecas, A. R. (1984). Regression of leiomyomata uteri following hypoestrogenism induced by repetitive luteinizing hormone agonist treatment: preliminary report. *Fertil. Steril.*, **42**, 644–6
31. Maheux, R., Lemay, A. and Merat, P. (1987). Use of intranasal luteinizing hormone-releasing hormone agonist in uterine leiomyomas. *Fertil. Steril.*, **47**, 229–33
32. Linder, C. H., Braendle, W., Bispink, L., Lichtenberg, V. and Bettendorf, G. (1987). Gonadotropin Simulation und *In vitro* Fertilization nach selektiver Hypophysen-Suppression durch LHRH Analogon. *Geburtsh. Frauenheilk.*, **47**, 490–4
33. Rutherford, A. J., Subak Sharpe, R. J., Dawson, K. J., Margara, R. A., Franks, S. and Winston, R. L. M. (1988). Improvement of *in vitro* fertilisation after treatment with Buserelin, an agonist of luteinising hormone releasing hormone. *Br. Med. J.*, **296**, 1765–8
34. Kupesic, S. and Kurjak, A. (1993). Uterine and ovarian perfusion during the periovulatory period assessed by transvaginal color Doppler. *Fertil. Steril.*, **60**, 439–43
35. Glissant, A., de Mouzon, J. and Frydman, R. (1985). Ultrasound study of the endometrium during *in vitro* fertilization cycles. *Fertil. Steril.*, **44**, 786–90

Benign uterine conditions: what does color add?

12

A. Kurjak and S. Kupesic

Color and pulsed Doppler can add important diagnostic information in different benign uterine conditions.

UTERINE ABNORMALITIES

Direct visualization of the uterine vasculature, which is displayed simultaneously with the conventional B-mode image, allows fast and accurate velocimetry of the uterine arteries in normal volunteers and patients with congenital uterine anomalies. Kurjak and Kupesic[1] evaluated uterine perfusion in 34 patients with duplication anomalies of the uterus (26 bicornuate and eight uterus didelphys). No difference was detected ($p > 0.05$) in uterine artery blood flow during the early proliferative phase of the menstrual cycle between these two groups of patients (Table 1).

Uterine fibroids or leiomyomas

Transvaginal sonography with color flow imaging facilitates the measurement of blood flow impedance in small vascular branches and increases the reproducibility of the measurements[2,3]. Small vessels that feed growing leiomyomas[4,5] and uterine blood flow patterns[6–11] can easily be detected by this method (Color plate I). Vascularization of benign uterine masses is supported by normal existing vessels. When color flow is present, waveform analysis indicates blood flow impedance as slighty decreased or similar to the normal myometrial perfusion originating from terminal branches of the uterine artery. Diastolic flow is always present in premenopausal patients, and is usually increased in comparison with the uterine artery blood flow (Color plate J). Color flow detects the myoma's feeder vessels that arise from the myometrial vasculature and form a regular ring of angiogenesis, and central vessels that develop as a response to the angiogenic activity of tumor cells, perhaps due to necrotic and inflammatory processes.

The mean Pourcelot resistance index (RI) of myometrial blood flow is 0.54, and the mean pulsatility index (PI) is 0.89. Very low resistance indices are usually present in cases with necrosis and secondary degenerative and inflammatory changes within the fibroid (Color plate K). The same technique was used to study uterine artery blood flow in patients with uterine fibroids and healthy volunteers attending our Ultrasonic Institute for their annual check-up[5]. Increased blood flow velocity and decreased RI and PI in both uterine arteries occurred in patients with uterine fibroids (Table 2). The difference in the vascular signatures noted in this study may have predictive value in growth rate evaluation of these benign uterine masses.

Transvaginal color Doppler sonography seems to be helpful in identifying vascularized myomas responsive to gonadotropin hormone analog treatment[8], and in optimizing the timing of surgery. A particularly interesting observation was made in postmenopausal patients with fibroids that regressed after menopause. The blood flow detected on the periphery of the fibroids showed a different pattern (higher RI) from that observed in premenopausal patients, sometimes even presenting the absence of end-diastolic flow. Furthermore, this non-invasive diagnostic tool can be used for studying iatrogenic effects on uterine morphology and perfusion. This may precisely answer the question of whether hormonal replacement therapy increases the risk of myometrial neoplasia.

Table 1 Uterine artery flow velocity in a group of fertile women ($n=30$) and infertile patients with congenital uterine anomalies ($n=34$). Values are shown ±standard deviation (original data)

	Control group ($n=30$)	*Bicornuate uterus* ($n=24$)	*Duplex uterus* ($n=18$)
Maximum peak systolic velocity (cm/s)			
Right uterine artery	28.23±8.14	30.49±8.50	29.64±7.16
Left uterine artery	28.98±8.48	32.02±8.02	32.64±7.02
Resistance index			
Right uterine artery	0.84±0.09	0.82±0.08	0.83±0.08
Left uterine artery	0.86±0.08	0.85±0.07	0.85±0.08
Pulsatility index			
Right uterine artery	2.52±0.87	2.38±0.82	2.42±0.87
Left uterine artery	2.68±0.87	2.64±0.87	2.60±0.92

Table 2 Some characteristics of blood flow in uterine arteries in 101 patients with palpable (avascularized, column 2; and vascularized, column 3) uterine fibroids and 60 healthy women (column 1). All examinations were performed in days 5–8 of the menstrual cycle

	Controls ($n=60$)	*Avascularized fibroids* ($n=30$)	*Vascularized fibroids* ($n=71$)	*p-values (columns)*		
				1–2	*2–3*	*1–3*
Velocity (cm/s)	33.40±12.25	44.80±17.10	47.08±18.46	<0.001	>0.005	<0.05
Resistance index	0.84±0.09	0.80±0.10	0.74±0.09	<0.001	<0.001	>0.05
Pulsatility index	2.52±0.87	2.17±0.32	1.65±0.49	<0.001	<0.001	>0.05

The same method is helpful in differentiating intraligamentary fibroids from solid ovarian tumors. Within or on the periphery of the uterine mass, even when it is out of the contour of the uterus, it is possible to detect waveform signals that are typical for the uterine vascular network. Blood flow is usually similar to normal myometrial perfusion originating from the terminal branches of the uterine artery. On the other hand, small vessels that feed a growing adnexal tumor are of ovarian origin.

Because myomas are hormonally responsive, they usually grow during early pregnancy[12,13]. Kurjak and colleagues[15] and Kupesic-Urek and colleagues[16] studied hemodynamic changes in the maternal and fetal vascular components of the placenta in both early normal pregnancy and pregnancy associated with uterine fibroids[14,15]. No significant difference in the vascular impedance of blood flow between the observed groups was found ($p>0.05$). Uterine fibroids do not influence the hemodynamics of uteroplacental circulation, or the maternal or fetal components of the placental circulation[16]. The only noted difference was the increased blood velocity of the radial arteries ($p<0.001$, from the 10th to the 13th gestational week), probably due to the increased metabolism of fibroid cells.

The presence of the fibroid may produce venous dilatation, with consequent congestion of the myometrium and endometrium. In such circumstances, the uterine environment is not conducive to nidation of a fertilized egg, and the blood supply to a developing fetus might be inadequate[1]. Menorrhagia associated with leiomyomas is a possible consequence of congestion and dilatation of the subjacent endometrial venous plexuses by impinging on the inner radial and arcuate veins.

ADENOMYOSIS

Increased myometrial perfusion (mean RI$=0.56$) can be detected from the periphery of the endometrial clusters which are usually localized adjacent to the endometrium[1] (Table 3). In severe cases, endometrial tissue extends through the myometrium and even penetrates the serosa. In such cases, areas of hemorrhage and clots within the muscle, together with dilated myometrial vessels, cause a 'Swiss cheese' appearance of

Table 3 Transvaginal color Doppler in the assessment of benign uterine masses ($n=250$) (original data)

Histopathology	*n*	*Color flow* *n*	*Color flow* *%*	*Resistance index (mean ± SD)*
Leiomyoma	151	106	70.2	0.54 ± 0.09
Adenomyosis	65	43	66.2	0.54 ± 0.12
Endometriotic cyst	4	1	25.0	0.58
Endometrial hyperplasia	17	11	64.7	0.50 ± 0.07
Endometrial polyp	13	6	46.2	0.48 ± 0.06

the myometrium. The RI of the uterine arteries shows a decrease (mean RI = 0.75), depending on the severity of the case (Color plate L).

ENDOMETRIUM

Transvaginal color Doppler permits simultaneous visualization of the endometrium and its vascular network under physiological and pathophysiological conditions. Endometrial perfusion may be helpful in distinguishing the etiology of abnormal endometrial thickening.

Secretory phase of the menstrual cycle

The hystological pattern of secretory endometrium includes a remarkably increased vascularization. During the ovulatory cycle, there is a sharp increase in end-diastolic velocities of the endometrial blood flow between the proliferative and secretory phases of the menstrual cycle. These changes might reflect the anticipated reception and maintenance of a blastocyst[15].

Decidua

When the uterine cavity is empty, showing a decidual reaction or only a weak central fluid ring, a suspicion of ectopic pregnancy has to be aroused if the pregnancy test is positive. The specific ultrasonic demonstration of ectopic pregnancy is limited to the cases with clear visualization of a living embryo or a gestational ring outside the uterus. When a non-specific complex adnexal mass is present, transvaginal color Doppler is helpful in demonstrating low impedance flow on the side of ectopia[17].

In contrast to the two concentric rings of decidua identified in early intrauterine pregnancy, the decidual ring associated with ectopic pregnancy has only one layer of decidua. Jurkovic and colleagues[18] compared the vascular signature in these two conditions. They found that blood flow impedance in uterine and spiral arteries, and corpus luteum blood vessels, showed no significant difference between intrauterine and ectopic pregnancies. Peak systolic velocity in the uterine arteries precisely reflected an increased blood supply on the side of ectopic gestation.

Endometritis

This condition may produce increased thickness, echogenicity and vascularity of the endometrium and inner third of myometrium[19] (Color plate M). The waveforms detected from such color-coded areas showed a moderately high resistance index (RI > 0.50).

Endometrial hyperplasia

Endometrial thickness greater than 14 mm in premenopausal women and greater than 8 mm in postmenopausal women, should be an indicator for further investigation. Endometrial thickness, morphology and integrity of the subendometrial halo are factors that can accurately be used to distinguish endometrial pathology from normal endometrium. However, morphology itself can not be used to discriminate benign from malignant conditions. Color and pulsed Doppler features serve as additional discriminative criteria for more accurate diagnosis of endometrial pathology. A significant difference has been found in terms of the RI value between endometrial malignancy (mean RI = 0.42) and endometrial hyperplasia (mean RI = 0.50) (Table 3). Furthermore, the peripheral distribution of the regularly separated vessels is typical of endometrial hyperplasia (Color plate N), while the 'dense' vascular arrangement is pathognomonic for malignancy.

Endometrial polyps

The vascularization of endometrial polyps is supported by already existing vessels (Color plate O), originating from terminal branches of the uterine arteries[1,19] (Table 3). Those polyps that are secondarily changed (necrosis and inflammation) usually show alterations in endometrial perfusion. A marked reduction in blood flow impedance noted on the periphery and/or within the endometrial polyps may lead an inexperienced ultrasonographer to false-positive diagnosis of endometrial malignancy.

Adhesions

Endometrial irregularities or hyperechoic bridges within the endometrial cavity that can be precisely outlined during menstruation, or following distention of the uterine cavity with fluid, do not present increased vascularity[1].

Intrauterine contraceptive device

Transvaginal sonography is very precise in the detection of malposition of an intrauterine contraceptive device, its partial myometrial invasion or its incomplete removal. Color Doppler facilities are also helpful in detecting acute pelvic inflammatory disease (Color plate M) and ectopic pregnancy, the development of which is increased in patients with such a device[1].

CERVIX

Nabothian cysts are visualized as small, thin-walled cystic structures near the endocervical canal, and usually do not demonstrate increased vascularity. In cases with clear vascular signals, pulsed Doppler waveform analysis demonstrates low-velocity and high-impedance flow (Color plate P). Cervical pregnancy is a rare condition that may be misinterpreted as cervical inclusion cyst. The waveforms obtained from the periphery of such a structure show low impedance signals very similar to the vascularity of early intrauterine gestation.

References

1. Kurjak, A. and Kupesic, S. (1994). Benign uterine conditions. In Kurjak, A. (ed.) *An Atlas of Transvaginal Color Doppler*, pp. 247–317. (Carnforth, UK: Parthenon Publishing)
2. Hata, T., Hata, K. and Senoch, D. (1989). Transvaginal Doppler flow mapping. *Gynecol. Obstet. Invest.*, **27**, 217
3. Kurjak, A. and Zalud, I. (1991). The characterization of uterine tumors by transvaginal color Doppler. *Ultrasound Obstet. Gynecol.*, **1**, 50–2
4. Shimamoto, K., Sakuma, S., Ishigaki, T. and Makino, N. (1987). Intratumoral blood flow: evaluation with color Doppler echography. *Radiology*, **165**, 683–5
5. Kurjak, A., Kupesic-Urek, S. and Miric, D. (1992). The assessment of benign uterine tumor vascularization by transvaginal color Doppler. *Ultrasound Med. Biol.*, **18**, 645–8
6. Goswamy, R. K. and Steptoe, P. C. (1988). Doppler ultrasound studies of the uterine artery in spontaneous ovarian cycles. *Hum. Reprod.*, **3**, 721–6
7. Kurjak, A., Kupesic-Urek, S., Schulman, H. and Zalud, I. (1991). Transvaginal color Doppler in the assessment of ovarian and uterine perfusion in infertile women. *Fertil. Steril.*, **6**, 870–3
8. Matta, W. M., Stabile, I., Shaw, R. W. and Campbell, S. (1988). Doppler assessment of uterine blood flow changes in patients with fibroids receiving the gonadotropin-releasing hormone agonist Buserelin. *Fertil. Steril.*, **49**, 1083–5
9. Sholtes, M. C. W., Wladimiroff, J. W., van Rijen, H. J. M. and Hop, W. C. J. (1989). Uterine and ovarian flow velocity waveforms in the normal menstrual cycle: a transvaginal color Doppler study. *Fertil. Steril.*, **53**, 981–5
10. Kurjak, A., Zalud, I., Jurkovic, D., Alfirevic, Z. and Miljan, M. (1989). Transvaginal color Doppler for the assessment of pelvic circulation. *Acta Obstet. Gynecol. Scand.*, **68**, 131–5
11. Kurjak, A., Jurkovic, D., Alfirevic, Z. and Zalud, I. (1990). Transvaginal color Doppler imaging. *J. Clin. Ultrasound*, **18**, 227–31

12. Lev-Toaff, A. S., Coleman, B. G. and Arger, P. H. (1987). Leiomyomas in pregnancy: sonographic study. *Radiology*, **164**, 375–80
13. Rosati, P., Bellatti, U. and Exacoustos, C. (1989). Uterine myoma in pregnancy: ultrasound study. *Int. J. Gynaecol. Obstet.*, **28**, 109–17
14. Kurjak, A., Kupesic-Urek, S. and Miric, D. (1991). Transvaginal color Doppler in the assessment of uterine blood flow changes during the pregnancy in patients with fibroids. *J. Perinat. Med.*, **19** (Suppl. 2), 81
15. Kupesic-Urek, S. and Kurjak, A. (1991). Transvaginal color Doppler in the assessment of uterine artery blood flow in early pregnancy complicated by uterine mass. *J. Matern. Fetal. Invest.*, **1**, 163
16. Kurjak, A., Predanic, M., Kupesic-Urek, S., Zudenigo, D., Matijevic, R. and Salihagic, A. (1991). Transvaginal color Doppler in the study of early normal pregnancies and pregnancies associated with uterine fibroids. *J. Matern. Fetal. Invest.*, **2**, 81–5
17. Kurjak, A., Zalud, I. and Schulman, H. (1991). Ectopic pregnancy: transvaginal color Doppler of trophoblastic flow in questionable adnexa. *J. Ultrasound Med.*, **10**, 685–9
18. Jurkovic, D., Bourne, T., Jauniaux, E., Campbell, S. and Collins, P. W. (1992). Transvaginal color Doppler study of blood flow in ectopic pregnancy. *Fertil. Steril.*, **57**, 68–73
19. Kurjak, A. and Kupesic-Urek, S. (1992). Normal and abnormal uterine perfusion. In Jaffe, R. and Warsof, S. (eds.) *Color Doppler Imaging*, p. 225. (New York: McGraw-Hill)

Malignant uterine tumors 13

A. Kurjak and S. Kupesic

In the first part of this book, much important information on the role of ultrasound in the diagnosis of malignant pathology of the uterus is described in detail. It is the purpose of this chapter to evaluate the role of color and pulsed Doppler in this important area.

There have been several reports[1–5] on the role of transvaginal color and pulsed Doppler sonography in detecting gynecological malignancies. The distinction between benign and malignant conditions is based on the detection of tumoral vessels that exhibit low impedance and high diastolic blood flow[6] and the process of tumor angiogenesis, which is necessary for tumor growth[7]. The newly formed vessels are recognized microscopically by the lack of smooth muscle in their intima, combined with arteriovenous shunting that occurs within the neoplasm[8,9].

In this chapter, we discuss the value of transvaginal color Doppler in early detection of endometrial cancer and the role of color Doppler ultrasonography in determining the depth of myometrial penetration and tumor staging whenever invasion is suspected. Furthermore, we evaluate the role of this method in differentiating uterine sarcoma from myoma, as well as its possible application in the diagnosis and follow-up of patients with cervical carcinoma.

ENDOMETRIAL CARCINOMA

Recent color Doppler studies[6,10–14] have attempted to improve sensitivity and specificity of transvaginal sonography for diagnosing endometrial carcinoma. Color and pulsed Doppler features express the tumor's vascular nature, which can be used as an additional criterion for evaluation of endometrial morphology, for more accurate diagnosis of endometrial malignancy.

Although uterine bleeding is the most common initial symptom of endometrial cancer, only 10% of women with postmenopausal bleeding have endometrial cancer.

Sclerotic changes of the vessels with consequent venous or arterial rupture are shown in the majority of women with postmenopausal bleeding[15]. However, this bleeding can be caused by benign uterine conditions, such as endometrial hyperplasia, endometrial polyps or submucous myomas[16].

Till now, dilatation and curettage has been used as the 'gold standard' for detection of endometrial carcinoma[16]. Some studies[16–18] showed that areas of endometrial neoplasia could easily be missed in 2–6% of cases. Therefore, the use of color flow imaging, added to conventional two-dimensional transvaginal sonography, may become a non-invasive method of choice for investigation of endometrial abnormalities[19].

A transvaginal color and pulsed Doppler study performed in our Department[6] evaluated 750 hysterectomized postmenopausal women for different gynecological indications. Thirty-five cases with endometrial carcinoma were diagnosed histologically, and 32 of them (91%) were detected by transvaginal color Doppler ultrasonography. Of the cases with detected endometrial carcinoma, 90% had endometrial thickness of over 10 mm (usually > 20 mm); 10% of cases with endometrial carcinoma showed thickness ranging from 5 to 10 mm. Endometrial thickness of < 5 mm was consistent with 100% of atrophic and 70% of normal endometrium; there were no cases of endometrial cancer among these. In this group, we were not able to detect any arterial endometrial blood flow (Figure 1).

Endometrial carcinoma was diagnosed mostly by hyperechoic (45%) or inhomogeneous (45%) echo texture; only 10% had a hypoechoic pattern when compared with myometrium (Figure 2).

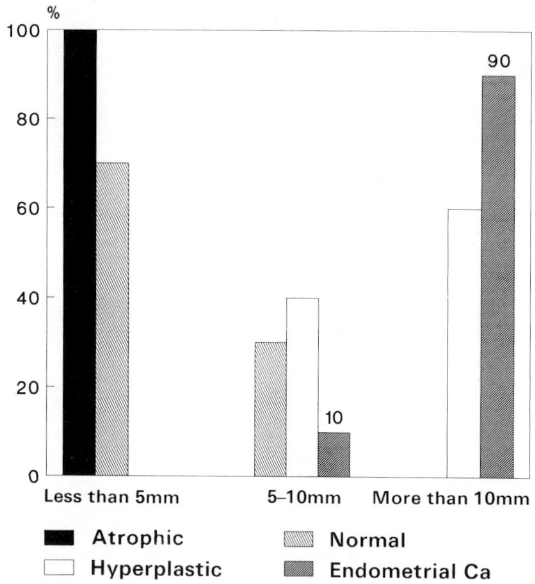

Figure 1 Endometrial thickness correlated with histopathological results in the endometrium. Most of the endometrial carcinomas (90%) were >10 mm thick (reprinted with permission from reference 6)

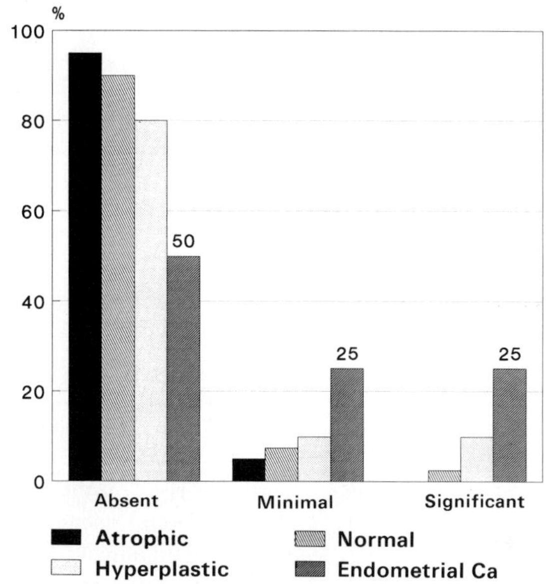

Figure 3 Presence of intracavitary fluid correlated with histopathological results in the endometrium. The presence of significant fluid was consistent with endometrial carcinoma (reprinted with permission from reference 6)

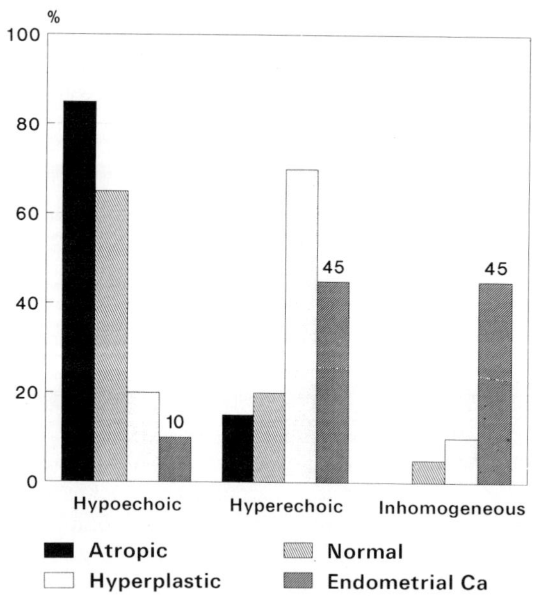

Figure 2 Echogenicity of the endometrium corrected with histopathological results in the endometrium. Most of the endometrial carcinomas were hyperechogenic or inhomogeneous in relation to the myometrium (reprinted with permission from reference 6)

The presence of significant intrauterine fluid was consistent with endometrial carcinoma in most of the cases (Figure 3). However, the absence of intracavitary fluid did not exclude malignancy. A subendometrial halo was visualized in 90% of detected endometrial carcinomas, while the presence of interrupted halo was consistent with myometrial invasion (Figure 4). The depth of myometrial invasion was evaluated in three cases as superficial (invading less than half of the myometrial thickness) and in 15 cases as deep (invading more than half of the myometrial thickness) (Table 1).

Endometrial arterial blood flow was absent in normal, atrophic and 92% of hyperplastic endometria. In 91% of endometrial carcinomas, intratumoral or peritumoral blood flow was displayed (Table 2). The mean resistance index (RI) obtained from visualized vessels was 0.42 ± 0.02 (Color plate Q). The peak systolic velocities recorded in these vessels were relatively high; for intratumoral vessels, the mean velocity was 12.04 ± 3.1 cm/s, whereas that of peritumoral vessels was 17.12 ± 2.7 cm/s (Table 3). The differ-

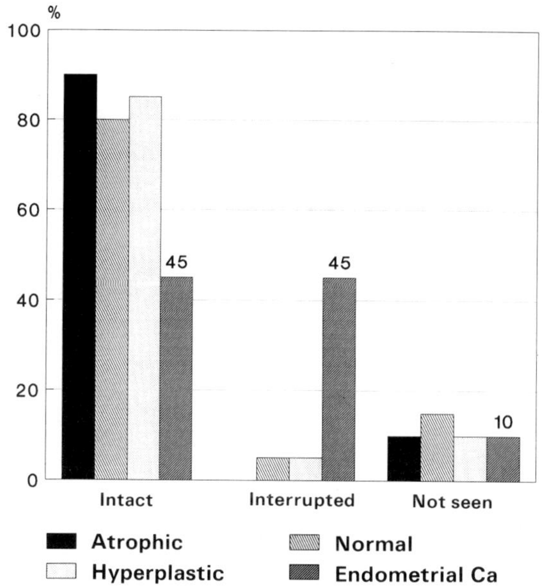

Figure 4 Integrity of subendometrial halo correlated with histopathological results in the endometrium. The halo was interrupted in cases of invasive endometrial carcinoma (reprinted with permission from reference 6)

ence between both velocities was statistically significant ($p<0.05$). Three asymptomatic women had endometrial carcinoma (two stage IA and one stage IB, by FIGO classification) detected. On B mode, thick (> 10 mm) inhomogeneous endometria with intact subendometrial halo were displayed. Color flow revealed areas of vascularization within the endometrial echo, Doppler waveform analysis showing low impedance to blood flow (RI < 0.42).

The conclusion of this study was that transvaginal color and pulsed Doppler sonography can depict endometrial carcinoma, even in asymptomatic women, determine the depth of myometrial invasion and help in tumor staging.

Merce and co-workers[9] studied 45 patients with metrorrhagia and compared their findings with those in 19 normal women. The authors used a duplex system with a transvaginal probe. They measured the Doppler signals in both uterine arteries and in the myometrium, which they assumed to be in the region of the radial and arcuate arteries. A significant decrease in the RI of the uterine and intramyometrial arteries was found in women with endometrial abnormalities.

Table 1 Ultrasonographic and pathological assessment of myometrial invasion in endometrial cancer (reprinted with permission from reference 6)

	Ultrasonographic	*Pathological*
Non-invasive	14	16
Invasive		
superficial	3	4
deep	15	15
Total	32*	35

*The three cases missed by ultrasonography were examined within 1 week after curettage

The authors concluded that the RI of the intramyometrial (arcuate and radial) arteries was highly accurate in predicting the positive findings, when compared to the RI of the uterine arteries, which was less accurate and less specific in predicting endometrial pathology.

Bourne and associates[10] studied uterine artery perfusion in patients with endometrial carcinoma and those with normal morphology of the uterus. They reported a significant difference in values of the pulsatility index (PI) between the groups and estimated a cut-off value of 2.00. The positive predictive value of this study was 80.9%, while the negative predictive value reached 99.9%. In their later publication[2], Bourne and associates reported an arbitrary cut-off value of 1.5 for uterine artery PI as a basis for a positive test result. They concluded that the predictive value of a positive test result in postmenopausal patients presenting with bleeding would be 94%. The predictive value might have been even higher if minor vessels had been selected.

It seems that the uterine artery itself is too large to show hemodynamic disturbances caused by a small area of neovascularization in the early stages of endometrial carcinoma. On the other hand, in the advanced stages, where specific vessels cannot be identified due to massive necrosis, the uterine artery blood flow shows a significant reduction in impedance.

Hata and colleagues[4] measured the RI in the arcuate arteries of 10 cases with endometrial carcinoma and in normal healthy women matched for age and parity. A significantly lower value was obtained from the arcuate artery wreath of patients with endometrial cancer (RI = 0.53 ± 0.15) than in controls

Table 2 Blood flow visualization and resistance index in relation to histopathological characteristics (reprinted with permission from reference 6)

		Flow visualization rate		*Resistance index*	
	n	*n*	%	*Mean*	*SD*
Atrophic	10	0	0	–	–
Normal	643	0	0	–	–
Hyperplastic	62	5	8	0.65*	0.05
Endometrial carcinoma	35	32	91	0.42*	0.02

*Statistically significant ($p<0.05$).
†Peak systolic velocity detected only in peritumoral vessels.

Table 3 Location of tumoral blood vessels, velocity, and resistance index in endometrial carcinoma (reprinted with permission from reference 6)

	Intratumoral ($n=22$)	*Peritumoral* ($n=28$)
Peak systolic velocity (cm/s)		
Mean	12.04*	17.12
SD	3.1	2.7
Resistance index		
Mean	0.39*	0.43
SD	0.03	0.03

*Statistically significant ($p<0.05$)

(RI$=0.76\pm0.17$). The same group[11] reported a 100% (9/9) visualization rate of feeder arteries and 77% (7/9) for intratumoral vessels. Intratumoral blood flow was characterized by low impedance of both arterial and venous signals. Intratumoral hemodynamic changes have been followed by the same technique[12] before and during hypertensive intra-arterial chemotherapy. The mean peak systolic velocity during hypertensive intra-arterial chemotherapy (58.9 ± 29.3 cm/s) was significantly higher than that before chemotherapy (16.0 ± 6.3) ($p<0.05$). Furthermore, there was a significant difference between the RI value during chemotherapy (0.61 ± 0.09) and before therapy (0.64 ± 0.12) ($p<0.05$). These results suggest that hypertensive intra-arterial chemotherapy induces a selective marked increase of blood flow in uterine cancer.

Bonilla and colleagues[13] reported a visualization rate of 97% for intratumoral blood vessels in 67 patients with histologically proved endometrial cancer. The authors concluded that sensitivity and specificity in the detection of endometrial adenocarcinomas were significantly increased by using color Doppler facilities than by using endometrial thickness depicted by transvaginal sonography alone. Rudigoz and Gaucherand[14] suggested the combination of morphological (endometrial/uterine thickness ratio) and Doppler criteria for detection of endometrial malignancy. An abnormal blood flow pattern was found in six out of seven endometrial cancers with the RI range from 0.47 to 0.60. Quite contrary results were published by Sladkevicius and Valentin[20]. They found that color Doppler analysis did not add any new information for discrimination between benign and malignant endometrial pathology.

Until now, curettage and histological evaluation have been necessary for definitive diagnosis[21]. However, the operation is relatively costly, carries a small but real risk of morbidity and causes a great deal of anxiety to the patient[22].

In contrast, transvaginal ultrasonography is a simple, non-invasive technique, highly accepted by patients[23]. The enhanced resolution afforded by the currently available transvaginal probes has significantly improved the ability of this technique to depict endometrial pathological features and the depth of myometrial invasion. Based on our experience[6], the features highly suggestive of endometrial carcinoma are endometrial thickness of >10 mm (20 ± 7 mm), inhomogeneous or hyperechoic endometrial echoes, and the presence of intrauterine fluid (Figures 1–4). Myometrial invasion was common when the subendometrial halo was interrupted (Figure 4). The impedance to blood flow in intratumoral and peritumoral vessels in endometrial cancer constituted a statisti-

Table 4 Blood flow characteristics in the detection of endometrial carcinoma

	Uterine artery		*Tumoral blood flow*	
Authors	*Mean RI*	*Mean PI*	*Mean RI*	*Mean PI*
Bourne *et al.*[2]	–	0.89	–	0.49
Bourne *et al.*[10]	–	0.91	–	–
Hata *et al.*[11]	0.53*	–	–	–
Hata *et al.*[12]	–	–	0.64	–
Kurjak *et al.*[6]	–	–	0.42	–
Zeitoun *et al.*[24]	0.81	1.82	0.52	0.62
Rudigoz *et al.*[14]	–	–	0.47–0.60	–

RI, resistance index; PI, pulsatility index; *, arcuate arteries

cally lower value with that of benign endometrial conditions ($p<0.05$). Moreover, intratumoral vessels displayed lower velocity compared with that of peritumoral blood vessels. It can be postulated that peritumoral vascularity develops as a direct response to the angiogenic activity of tumor cells and represents the area of extensive tumoral growth.

It should be stressed that three cases out of 95 patients were missed. In all of these, curettage was performed 1 week before color Doppler examination, which probably had altered endometrial hemodynamics. Therefore, transvaginal color Doppler should be performed before dilatation and curettage intervention. Three cases of endometrial carcinoma (two stage IA and one stage IB) were asymptomatic and revealed by color Doppler ultrasonography on the basis of the presence of thick endometrium (>20 mm) and the existence of intratumoral and/or peritumoral blood flow with a low RI (<0.42). In these cases, 'dense' vessel arrangement was observed.

Table 4 presents a review of color Doppler studies on endometrial carcinoma. Although different results in terms of RI and PI are presented, the message is that color and pulsed Doppler is a useful additional tool in differentiating benign from suspicious and malignant endometrial pathology, when enlarged thickness of the endometrium is observed in symptomatic or asymptomatic postmenopausal patients. Undoubtedly, this technique has a great potential in diagnosis and staging of endometrial carcinoma in high-risk groups. It is hoped that published results[6,10–14] will encourage the widespread use of this non-invasive technique, which will possibly result in a significant reduction of dilatation and curettage operations, with considerable savings of both the potential risks and economic costs.

During our 5-year study, 5013 asymptomatic women (44% premenopausal and 56% postmenopausal) were scanned by transvaginal color and pulsed Doppler ultrasonography in an attempt to detect malignancy[25]. Thirty-four (0.68%) cases of endometrial abnormalities were detected and operated on. Of these, six (0.12%) were endometrial carcinoma, 18 (0.36%) were endometrial hyperplasia, and 10 (0.20%) were benign endometrial polyps. These cases were brought to treatment and benefited well from the screening program.

The conclusion is that the application of transvaginal color Doppler sonography to the general population in order to screen for endometrial carcinoma may be a viable option if combined with ovarian screening in the same scan. In this way, the capital costs of the screening would be shared, and an oncological preventive medicine program for (postmenopausal) women would be created.

UTERINE SARCOMA

Another useful application of color and pulsed Doppler is possible in *in vivo* recognition of uterine sarcoma. This tumor is unique, because it is both rare and characterized by extremely aggressive behavior, which leads to an early pattern of widespread dissemination and death. It is expected to be more common in the near future, since gynecologists are gaining familiarity with

Table 5 Resistance index (RI) and peak-systolic velocity (Ps) in the myometrium of sarcomatous, myomatous and normal uteri

		Visualization rate		*Resistance index*		*Peak-systolic velocity*	
	n	*n*	*%*	*Mean*	*SD*	*Mean*	*SD*
Normal uterus	50	21	42	0.68	0.02	32.2	4.4
Myomatous uterus	50	34	61	0.54	0.08	28.4	7.3
Sarcomatous uterus	10	10	100	0.37	0.03	16.8	6.4

Table 6 Resistance index in both right and left uterine arteries in the studied groups

		Right artery		*Left artery*	
	n	*Mean*	*SD*	*Mean*	*SD*
Normal uterus	50	0.87	0.09	0.89	0.04
Myomatous uterus	50	0.74	0.08	0.75	0.08
Sarcomatous uterus	10	0.62	0.07	0.63	0.06

the conservative treatment of uterine myomas[26]. Therefore, any method that can accurately and non-invasively diagnose myometrial malignancy and differentiate it from common benign lesions is urgently required.

Our study (A. Kurjak and colleagues, unpublished) assessed blood flow indices of primary vessels (uterine artery) and secondary vessels (intratumoral neovascularization) in ten cases of uterine sarcoma. The typical finding in sarcoma was the presence of irregular, thin and randomly dispersed vessels in the peripheral and/or central area of the tumor, with very low impedance shunts. Furthermore, in the group of patients with sarcoma, both uterine arteries showed a low RI in comparison with that of normal or myomatous uteri in women matched for age and parity (Table 5). In the group of normal healthy vounteers, the uterine artery RI was around 0.88. Decreased values, such as 0.74 ($p<0.05$) were present in patients with uterine leiomyomas and 0.63 ($p<0.001$) in those with uterine sarcomas. There was no statistical difference ($p>0.05$) between the RI in the right and the left uterine arteries in each group separately (Table 6).

Color Doppler revealed areas of neovascularization (at the border or/and in the center of the tumor) in all patients with sarcoma (100%), while only 61% of myomas were vascularized. Diastolic flow was present in all the uterine lesions detected and was increased in comparison with the uterine artery blood flow. The mean RI in cases with sarcoma was 0.37 ± 0.03 (Color plate R) which constituted a statistically significant difference ($p<0.05$) from that of myomas (0.54 ± 0.08). The mean Pourcelot RI of myometrial blood flow in normal volunteers was 0.68 and was significantly higher ($p<0.05$) than the other two examined groups. Three women with leiomyosarcoma (stage I) were successfully detected by transvaginal color and pulsed Doppler (one during the prospective study).

Kurjak and colleagues[27] demonstrated that the vascularization of benign uterine masses is largely dependent on the tumor size, its position and the extent of secondary degenerative changes. Large and laterally positioned leiomyomas, especially those with necrosis and inflammatory changes, may show increased diastolic flow and consequently, a low RI. It seemed clear from conflicting Doppler data that differences and improvements in instrument design had made smaller vessels more visible. Visualization of smaller vessels has led to the recognition of occasional low-resistance vessels in benign growths. Biological variation dictates that all malignant growths might not have vessels, particularly if growth has stabilized or if there is no metastatic potential.

We have demonstrated an overlap between three cases of uterine myomas with uterine sarcomas in terms of an RI cut-off point of 0.40. This observation awaits further studies, as it could be due to the rapid rate of growth of such myomas or be due to a premalignant state. It can be postulated that leiomyomas arise *de novo* in most cases, but some are thought to arise from malignant transformation of a pre-existing leiomyoma. In many cases, gross pathology cannot distinguish leiomyosarcoma from leiomyoma with degeneration and irregular borders. Sometimes, only a high mitotic count is important in distinguishing sarcomas from cellular myomas[28,29].

During a 1-year prospective study in our Department, transvaginal color Doppler detected one uterine sarcoma with low RI value (RI = 0.33), which fell into a borderline category. Microscopic pathology detected five mitoses per high-powered field (HPF) and moderate cellular atypia. Other sarcomas were characterized by moderate-to-marked cellular atypia and a mitotic rate in excess of 10 mitotic figures or 10/HPF. Moreover, some myomas show infiltration of the myometrium and cellular pleomorphism, albeit usually not to the degree seen in leiomyosarcoma. Therefore, careful transvaginal color Doppler examination of a uterine tumor should include morphological changes and analysis of vascularization (brightness of color, vascular location and type of vascularization). Malignant uterine masses display bright color signals from randomly dispersed vessels, while pulsed Doppler analysis demonstrates low vascular impedance (mean RI = 0.37 ± 0.03).

In very large and necrotic leiomyomas, areas of neovascularization within the central parts usually demonstrate low vascular impedance, due to release of vasoactive compounds, while the peripheral ring of angiogenesis is characterized by moderate impedance to blood flow. It seems that uterine artery peak systolic velocity and vascular impedance quality measured by RI or PI can be used as additional parameters in the diagnosis of leiomyosarcoma, since they showed significantly lower values when compared to those of uterine leiomyoma.

Weiner and co-workers[30] reported one case of stage III malignant uterine leiomyoblastoma. A multi-parameter score, which included transvaginal sonography, color flow imaging, computed tomography scan and serum CA 125 level, was positive for malignancy.

There are still many problems in distinguishing benign from malignant tumors *in vivo*. The gold standard is still histopathological examination of tissue obtained surgically. Indeed, a non-invasive method that accurately provides *in vivo* differentiation between benign and malignant uterine masses can solve many clinical problems. In this light, transvaginal color and pulsed Doppler seems to have better potential than do other non-invasive methods of tissue characterization.

However, it is unrealistic to expect Doppler studies to clarify confounding histological findings. A multi-parameter sonographic approach that includes morphology and size depicted by transvaginal ultrasonography and color flow imaging with pulsed Doppler analysis of neovascular signals can help in diagnosis of uterine sarcoma in high-risk groups, such as postmenopausal patients with rapidly enlarging uterus. Vascular location and type of tumoral vascularization should be determined along with the analysis of Doppler signal quality. Needless to say, experience of the examiner, both clinical and ultrasonic, is of paramount importance here.

CERVICAL CARCINOMA

The first explanation of why color and pulsed Doppler is less promising in detection of cervical malignancy is that efficacious diagnostic and screening methods already exist. Another is that the visualization of cervical malignancy may be difficult with transvaginal sonography, because the probe is too close to the cervix. An improvement in the visualization can be obtained by partly withdrawing the probe and angling it either posteriorly for anteverted uteri or anteriorly for retroverted uteri[31].

Hata and colleagues[32] studied the presence of neovascular signals in 36 patients with advanced cervical carcinoma using the transabdominal route. Abnormal blood flow signals were reported in only six (16.7%) cases, while absence of blood flow was noted in half (18/36) of the cases. In a later publication, the same group used the transvaginal approach[11]. In six out of seven patients with cervical carcinoma, it was possible to detect lower impedance signals (RI = 0.51 ± 0.09), which were significantly different from that of the main ascending branch of the uterine artery in controls ($RI = 0.88 \pm 0.04$).

In the recent publications from the Zagreb group[33,34], blood flow of both the ascending and the descending branch of the uterine artery was studied in healthy subjects and patients with cervical malignancy. In healthy volunteers, there was a significant difference in the maximum velocity, which was on average 12 cm/s in the descending branch and 37 cm/s in the ascending branch. The PI (average 3.1 ± 0.9) and the RI (0.86 ± 0.56) were not significantly different between the branches.

In 74 out of 89 patients with cervical carcinoma, it was possible to detect a lowered RI (average $RI = 0.57 \pm 0.14$) and PI (average $PI = 0.75 \pm 0.23$) compared to the normal controls (Color plate S). No difference was detected in terms of maximum blood flow velocity of the descending branch of the uterine artery between these two groups.

It seems that the stage of the disease changes the blood flow characteristics. Carcinoma *in situ* does not change the uterine artery blood flow, whereas stages I, II and III may enhance the local flow as a sign of fast growth. It was observed that advanced and necrotizing tumors have a relatively small blood supply relative to their overall size. Furthermore, the number of spots with detectable flow may be of diagnostic and prognostic value. In 36% of cases, there were one or two spots with measurable flow within the cervix, while 30% of patients showed more than four spots with measurable flow.

However, the major problem is that there is not yet a satisfactory ability to measure cervical blood flow in 17% of healthy women and patients with cervical malignancy. This means that, at this stage of diagnostic development, ultrasound with or without color Doppler is not suitable for screening purposes for cervical cancer.

References

1. Kurjak, A., and Zalud, I. (1991). The characterization of uterine tumors by transvaginal color Doppler. *Ultrasound Obstet. Gynecol.*, **1**, 50–2
2. Bourne, T. H., Campbell, S., Steer, C. V., Royston, P., Whitehead, M. I. and Collins, W. P. (1991). Detection of endometrial cancer by transvaginal ultrasonography with color flow imaging and blood flow analysis: a preliminary report. *Gynecol. Oncol.*, **40**, 253–9
3. Kurjak, A., Salihagic, A., Kupesic-Urek, S. and Predanic, A. (1992). Clinical value of the assessment of gynecological tumor angiogenesis by transvaginal color Doppler. *Ann. Med.*, **24**, 97–103
4. Hata, K., Makihara, K. and Hata, T. (1991). Transvaginal color Doppler imaging for hemodynamic assessment of reproductive tract tumors. *Jpn. Int. J. Gynecol. Obstet.*, **36**, 301–8
5. Kurjak, A., Schulman, H., Sosic, A. and Zalud, I. (1992). Transvaginal ultrasound, color flow, and Doppler waveform of the postmenopausal adnexal mass. *Obstet. Gynecol.*, **80**, 917–21
6. Kurjak, A., Shalan, H., Sosic, A., Benic, S., Zudenigo, D., Kupesic, S. and Predanic, M. (1993). Endometrial carcinoma in postmenopausal women: evaluation by transvaginal color Doppler ultrasonography. *Am. J. Obstet. Gynecol.*, **169**, 1597–1603
7. Folkman, J., Watson, J., Ingber, D. and Hanahan, D. (1989). Induction of angiogenesis during the transition from hyperplasia to neoplasia. *Nature (London)*, **339**, 58–61
8. Kurjak, A., Shalan, H., Kupesic, S., Predanic, M., Breyer, B. and Jukic, S. (1993). Transvaginal color Doppler sonography in the assessment of pelvic tumor vascularity. *Ultrasound Obstet. Gynecol.*, **3**, 1–19
9. Merce, L. T., Garcia, L. and De La Fuente, F. (1991). Doppler ultrasound assessment of endometrial pathology. *Acta Obstet. Gynecol. Scand.*, **70**, 525–30
10. Bourne, T. H., Campbell, S., Whitehead, M. I., Royston, P., Steer, C. V. and Collins, W. P. (1990). Detection of endometrial cancer in postmenopausal women by transvaginal ultrasonography and color flow imaging. *Br. Med. J.*, **301**, 369–74
11. Hata, K., Hata, T., Manabe, A., Makihara, K. and Kitao, M. (1992). New pelvic sonography for detection of endometrial carcinoma: a preliminary report. *Gynecol. Oncol.*, **45**, 179–84
12. Hata, K., Hata, T., Manabe, A. and Kitao, M. (1992). Transvaginal Doppler ultrasound assessment of intratumoral hemodynamic change before and during hypertensive intra-arterial chemotherapy for uterine cancer. *Obstet. Gynecol.*, **80**, 801–4

13. Bonilla, F., Ballesteros, A. and Ballesteros, M. J. (1993). Transvaginal color Doppler in the diagnosis of endometrial adenocarcinomas. *Ultrasound Obstet. Gynecol.*, **3** (Suppl. 2), 23
14. Rudigoz, R. C. and Gaucherand, P. (1993). Vaginal sonography and color Doppler in postmenopausal abnormalities. *Ultrasound Obstet. Gynecol.*, **3** (Suppl. 2), 42
15. Choo, Y., Mak, K., Hsu, C. and Wong, T. (1985). Postmenopausal uterine bleeding of nonorganic cause. *Obstet. Gynecol.*, **66**, 225–31
16. Stowall, T. G., Solomon, S. K. and Ling, F. W. (1989). Endometrial sampling prior to hysterectomy. *Obstet. Gynecol.*, **73**, 405–9
17. Bistoletti, P., Hjerpe, A. and Mollerstrom, G. (1988). Cytological diagnosis of endometrial cancer and preinvasive endometrial lesions. *Acta Obstet. Gynecol. Scand.*, **67**, 342–5
18. McKenzie, I. Z. and Bibby, J. G. (1978). Critical assessment of dilatation and curettage in 1029 women. *Lancet*, **332**, 566–8
19. Kupesic, S., Shalan, H. and Kurjak, A. (1993). Early detection of endometrial cancer by transvaginal color Doppler. *Eur. J. Obstet. Gynecol.*, **49**, 46–9
20. Sladkevicius, P. and Valentin, L. (1993). Transvaginal color Doppler examination of women with postmenopausal bleeding. *Ultrasound Obstet. Gynecol.*, **3** (Suppl. 1), 25
21. Schonfeld, A., Levavi, H. and Hirsch, M. (1990). Transvaginal sonography in postmenopausal women. *J. Clin. Ultrasound*, **18**, 350–8
22. Granberg, S., Wikland, K. and Karlsson, B. (1991). Endometrial thickness as measured by endovaginal ultrasonography for identifying endometrial abnormality. *Am. J. Obstet. Gynecol.*, **164**, 47–52
23. Nasri, M. N., Shepherd, J. H. and Setchell, S. L. (1991). The role of vaginal scan in measurement of endometrial thickness in postmenopausal women. *Br. J. Obstet. Gynaecol.*, **98**, 470–5
24. Zeitoun, K., Aleen, F., Calame, R. and Penissi, J. (1993). Doppler flow indices and vascular color distribution in malignant and hyperplastic endometrium. *Ultrasound Obstet. Gynecol.*, **3** (Suppl. 2), 188
25. Kurjak, A., Shalan, H., Kupesic, A., Kosuta, D., Sosic, A., Benic, S., Ilijas, M., Jukic, S. and Predanic, M. (1994). An attempt to screen asymptomatic women for ovarian and endometrial cancer with transvaginal color and pulsed Doppler sonography. *J. Ultrasound Med.*, **13**, 295–301
26. Meyer, W. R., Meyer, A. R. and Diamond, M. P. (1990). Unsuspected leiomyosarcoma: treatment with a gonadotropin-releasing hormone analogue. *Obstet. Gynecol.*, **75**, 529–34
27. Kurjak, A., Kupesic-Urek, S. and Miric, D. (1992). The assessment of benign uterine tumors by transvaginal color Doppler. *J. Ultrasound Med. Biol.*, **18**, 645–9
28. Burns, B., Curry, H. R. and Bell, M. E. A. (1979). Morphologic features of prognostic significance in uterine smooth muscle tumors: a review of eighty-four cases. *Am. J. Obstet. Gynecol.*, **135**, 109–13
29. Ezra, J., Fieds, S. and Kopolovic, J. (1988). Benign uterine leiomyoma suspected of sarcomatous change on an ultrasound scan and computerized tomography. *Arch. Gynecol. Obstet.*, **241**, 255–9
30. Weiner, Z., Beck, D. and Brandes, J. M. (1994). Transvaginal sonography, color flow imaging, computed tomographic scanning, and CA 125 as a routine follow-up examination in women with pelvic tumor: detection of recurrent disease. *J. Ultrasound Med.*, **13**, 37–41
31. Fleischer, A. C. and Keppler, D. M. (1992). Benign conditions of the uterus, cervix and endometrium. In Nyberg, D. A., Hill, L. M., Bohm-Velez, M. and Mendelson, E. B. (eds.) *Transvaginal Ultrasound*, pp. 38–60. (St Louis: Mosby Year Book)
32. Hata, T., Hata, K., Senoh, D., Makihara, K., Aoki, S., Takamiya, O. and Kitao, M. (1989). Doppler ultrasound assessment of tumor vascularity in gynecologic disorders. *J. Ultrasound Med.*, **8**, 309–14
33. Breyer, B., Despot, A., Predanic, M. and Judin, S. (1993). Characteristics of blood flow in cancer of the uterine cervix. *Ultrasound Obstet. Gynecol.*, **3**, 268–70
34. Breyer, B., Despot, A. and Kurjak, A. (1994). Blood flow in malignancy of the uterine cervix. In Kurjak, A. (ed.) *Atlas of Transvaginal Color Doppler*, pp. 329–33. (Carnforth, UK: Parthenon Publishing)

Congestion syndrome of the uterus 14

A. Kurjak and S. Kupesic

Pelvic pain is one of the commonest complaints among young and middle-aged women treated as gynecological outpatients. It is a symptom that is frequently difficult to treat satisfactorily, because often no organic cause for the pain can be found. Commonly, the physician diagnoses pelvic inflammatory disease, with the result that the woman may be given repeated courses of antibiotics whenever the pain recurs[1]. Pelvic pain for which no obvious pathological cause can be found is a common problem in gynecological clinics. A survey carried out by the Royal College of Obstetricians and Gynaecologists on nearly 21 000 laparoscopies found that in 11 000, the primary indication was pain. In Gillibrand's study[2], 63% of patients undergoing laparoscopy showed no pathology.

The study of Beard and co-workers[3] confirmed that pelvic varicosities with concomitant vascular stasis and congestion are consistently found in women with pelvic pain syndrome.

The venous system of the pelvis is formed by multiple unsupported thin-walled veins, with weak attachments between the adventitia and the supporting connective tissue. Unlike those in the leg, these veins lack valves and depend largely on the fascia for their support. These differences allow for the extraordinary increase in their thickness in pregnancy, but also make them particularly vulnerable. Therefore, multiparity, constitutional defects and erect posture would explain their persistent dilatation. The histology of the vessel walls of pelvic varicosities is similar to that of varicose veins elsewhere[4]. Kaupilla[5] summarized the histological changes as fibrosis of the tunica intima and media, muscular hypertrophy, and proliferation of the capillary endothelium.

Hughes and Curtis[6] found that dilated veins were more frequently present with increasing parity, but they concluded that the effect was not great enough to affect the interpretation of pelvic venograms.

There are three possible mechanisms of pelvic congestion. Varicose veins are thought to result from the effects of gravity and defective valves. The worsening of pelvic pain in the erect position in women with pelvic pain syndrome and the improvement on lying down support this concept.

The second possibility is that an abnormal increase in blood flow through a region with many arteriovenous connections could lead to a state of chronic pelvic venous dilatation. Taylor and Duncan[7,8] suggested that 'pelvic congestion is a disorder of the pelvic autonomic nervous system arising in psychiatrically predisposed individuals'. The pelvis, being the site of rapid changes in blood flow that accompany environmental stress, and having unsupported veins, may well be predisposed to varicosities. In many instances, women with pelvic pain syndrome have a history of emotional stress, commonly originating from childhood[1].

The third possibility is that pelvic varicosities may occur as a result of relaxation of the smooth muscle in the walls of the pelvic veins caused by some vasoactive substance as yet unidentified[3].

The syndrome demonstrates the presence of abdominal pain in the minor pelvis. It is more common in the right iliac fossa, although some patients complain of left-sided pain, and its 'moving' from one side to the other is quite typical. Changes in position or abdominal pressure alter the symptomatology[9]. Therefore, standing, walking or jumping make the pain worse, whereas lying down eases the pain. It tends to be accompanied by a 'polysymptomatic' picture in which backache and headache together with leukorrhea are common. Dysmenorrhea (68%) and dysfunctional bleeding (54%) are also very frequent.

With the beginning and progress of their illness, many of these women noted changes in the frequency, duration, or amount of flow. It is noteworthy that excessive flow was not often reported.

The pain, as it is in the breast, is not menstrual but characteristically premenstrual in its time of appearance. In some cases, it is simply an exaggeration of the constant suprapubic and back pain experienced throughout the cycle. In others, these symptoms appear a few days to a week before the onset of the period and are usually considerably relieved by the onset of bleeding[10].

The premenstrual sysmptoms are almost certainly based upon the premenstrual swelling of already passively congested organs, and the menstrual cramps upon the perception of contractions in a similarly excessively congested organ. Some of the patients report intermenstrual bleeding. The bleeding is usually slight in amount and is not related to the probable time of ovulation. This symptom seems to be the result of minute hemorrhage from the excessively congested endometrium or endocervix and is not hormone-conditioned 'intracyclic bleeding'. Furthermore, in most of the studies, the uterus was found by palpation to be enlarged[1,3,7–10].

The uteri observed at operation are enlarged, soft and deep purple in color, suggesting even to the operator the possibility of an early pregnancy[10].

Leukorrhea is another symptom commonly presented in patients suffering from pelvic congestion syndrome. However, the discharge is always characterized by clear mucus, convincing evidence that it is due to a hypersecretion uncomplicated by infection.

The symptomatology can be frequently confused with polycystic ovarian syndrome or pelvic inflammatory disease. The description of the ovaries, parametria, breasts and peritoneum is beyond the scope of this chapter and can be found elsewhere[1,3,5,7–10].

The relative sterility in patients suffering from pelvic congestion may have its basis in several parts of the reproductive tract[10]. Endocervicitis offers a possible bar to the migration of sperm. The congested endometrium may afford an unfavorable ground for nidation. The tubes may be swollen or their folds agglutinated, a possibility suggested by the reaction of several cases to insufflation. Finally, ovarian function may be disturbed, either temporarily by congestion or permanently by the process of fibrosis.

Many methods have been employed to diagnose pelvic arteriovenous malformations, such as contrast-enhanced computed tomography and nuclear magnetic resonance[11], angiography[12], ultrasound and color Doppler sonography[13,14]. However, laparoscopy remains an essential part of the investigation of pelvic pain, because it is still the only reliable means of excluding endometriosis.

Procedures such as cervical dilatation and curettage and needle aspiration should be avoided, because of the potential for massive hemorrhage that would accompany any trauma to the arteriovenous malformations inadvertently caused by surgical instruments.

Pelvic venography has proved to be an invaluable research tool[15]. Although venography is an invasive and complicated procedure, it can be used with outpatients, giving them the opportunity to observe the dilated veins on the television monitor. However, this method does not provide complete 'vascular flow mapping', since it shows only the venous network[9]. In spite of being an excellent diagnostic technique, phlebography is less specific in the visualization of non-frequent locations (e.g. intrauterine involvement) or advanced congestive disease.

It is well known that mixed congestion does not always show a uniform vascular map. Therefore, it is possible to observe a predominantly venous component on one side, while arterial vessels missed by phlebography are located on the other side. Undoubtedly, this method has limitations (such as discomfort to the patients and inadequate diagnostic potential) and should not be used in a routine way.

The sonographic findings of pelvic arteriovenous malformations were first described by Torres and colleagues[16] and Diwan and associates[13]. Their findings included multiple serpentine, anechoic structures within the pelvis. Although real-time sonography depicts this feature, the findings of multiple cystic lesions in the pelvis suggest the occurrence of other entities as well, including hydrosalpinx, multilocular ovarian cysts, or fluid-filled loops of bowel. The diagnosis of pelvic arteriovenous malformations by means of transabdominal color Doppler flow imaging has been described recently by Musa and co-workers[17]. The differential diagnosis can be resolved with duplex and color Doppler applications.

Here, we discuss our unpublished results on 78 patients undergoing laparoscopy because of pelvic pain. This was a group with pelvic congestion syndrome and in whom no other concomitant pelvic pathology was found. The day before surgery, all were examined by transvaginal color and pulsed Doppler, which was decisive in diagnosis. In this short review, we concentrate on the uterus and its vascular network alone. The findings on vaginal examination showed uterine enlargement in 35 (44.9%) patients, while transvaginal sonography showed enlarged uterus in 70.5% of patients. Tenderness during bimanual compression of the uterus was reported in 71.8% of patients.

Furthermore, 75.9% of the women with pelvic congestion believed they had recurrent pelvic inflammatory disease. In 43.6% of patients with acute attacks, we were able to demonstrate dilatation of the intramyometrial vessels (Color plate T). The arterial type of uterine congestion caused predominantly acute symptoms, while the venous kind of congestion developed in patients with chronic pain.

Based on our experience, transvaginal color Doppler was shown as the safest and most definitive diagnostic technique within the gynecologist's reach, in this particular group of patients. To date, this technique has not been described frequently[18], but none the less opens an exceptional field for the future, because it allows arteries and veins to be distinguished. Its use has allowed a demonstration of the existence of vascular dilatation that affects not only the veins but also the arterial system. Sometimes, both systems are affected, with the vascular disturbance being much more intense and more widespread than described so far, because even the myometrial vessels can be affected (Figure 1, Color plate U). Therefore, cross sections of the dilated intramyometrial vessels may be misinterpreted as the 'Swiss cheese' appearance of the myometrium, as in a case of adenomyosis.

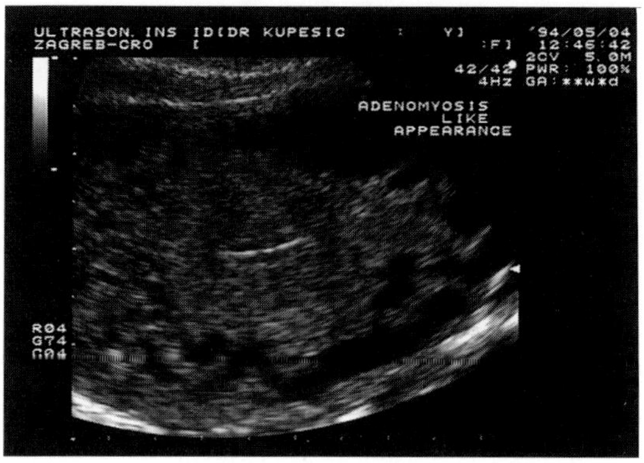

Figure 1 'Swiss cheese' appearance of the myometrium, common in patients suffering from adenomyosis

In conclusion, the visualization of the pelvic vessels with color Doppler allows us to differentiate the arterial from the venous component and to detect vascular alterations both at the peripheral level and at the intrauterine level. The venous plexuses are thick and in most cases observable with vaginal endosonography. This is not true for the arteries, which are much thinner. The arteries have a tendency to show their dilatation in intraparenchymatous locations and are usually visible only after color lighting of the vascular network.

References

1. Beard, R. W., Belsey, E. M., Leiberman, B. A. and Wilkinson, J. C. M. (1977). Pelvic pain in women. *Am. J. Obstet. Gynecol.*, **128**, 566–70
2. Gillibrand, P. N. (1981). The investigation of pelvic pain. Communication at the scientific meeting on *Chronic Pelvic Pain; a Gynaecological Headache*, Royal College of Obstetricians and Gynaecologists, London, May
3. Beard, R. W., Highman, J. H., Pearce, S. and Reginald, P. W. (1985). Diagnosis of pelvic varicosities in women with chronic pelvic pain. *Lancet*, **2**, 946–9

4. Renaer, M., Nijs, P., Van Assche, A. and Vertomman, H. (1980). Chronic pelvic pain without obvious pathology in women. Personal observations and a review of the problem. *Eur. J. Obstet. Gynecol. Reprod. Biol.*, **10**, 415–63
5. Kaupilla, A. (1970). Uterine phlebography with venous compression. A clinical and roentological study. *Acta Obstet. Gynecol. Scand.*, **49**, 33–4
6. Hughes, R. R. and Curtis, D. D. (1962). Uterine phlebography: correlation of clinical diagnoses with dye retention. *Am. J. Obstet. Gynecol.*, **83**, 156–64
7. Taylor, H. C. (1954). Pelvic pain based on a vascular and autonomic nervous system disorder. *Am. J. Obstet. Gynecol.*, **67**, 1177–96
8. Duncan, C. H. and Taylor, H. C. (1952). A psychosomatic study of pelvic congestion. *Am. J. Obstet. Gynecol.*, **64**, 1–12
9. Bonilla-Musoles, F. and Ballesteros, M. J. (1994). Transvaginal color Doppler in the diagnosis of pelvic congestion syndrome. In Kurjak, A. (ed.) *An Atlas of Transvaginal Color Doppler*, pp. 207–15. (Carnforth, UK: Parthenon Publishing)
10. Taylor, H. C. (1949). The clinical aspects of the congestion–fibrosis syndrome. *Am. J. Obstet. Gynecol.*, **57**, 637–53
11. Fakhri, A., Fisherman, E. K., Mitchell, S. E., Siegelman, S. S. and White, R. I. (1987). The role of CT in the management of pelvic arteriovenous malformations. *Cardiovasc. Intervent. Radiol.*, **10**, 96–9
12. Bottomley, J. P. and Whitehouse, G. H. (1975). Congenital arteriovenous malformations of the uterus demonstrated by angiography. *Acta Radiol.*, **16**, 43–8
13. Diwan, R. V., Brennan, J. N., Selim, M. A. *et al.* (1983). Sonographic diagnosis of arteriovenous malformations of the uterus and pelvis. *J. Clin. Ultrasound*, **11**, 295–8
14. Juhasq, B., Kurjak, A. and Lampe, L. G. (1992). Pelvic varices simulating bilateral adnexal masses: differential diagnosis by vaginal color Doppler. *J. Clin. Ultrasound*, **20**, 81–4
15. Beard, R. W., Reginald, P. W. and Wadsworth, J. (1988). Clinical features of women with chronic lower abdominal pain and pelvic congestion. *Br. J. Obstet. Gynaecol.*, **95**, 153–61
16. Torres, W. E., Stones, P. J. Jr and Thames, F. M. (1979). Ultrasound appearance of pelvic arteriovenous malformation. *J. Clin. Ultrasound*, **7**, 383–5
17. Musa, A. A., Hata, T., Hata, K. and Kitao, M. (1989). Pelvic arteriovenous malformation diagnosed by color flow Doppler imaging. *Am. J. Radiol.*, **152**, 1311–12
18. Jain, K. A., Jeffrey, R. B. and Sommer, F. G. (1991). Gynaecologic vascular abnormalities: diagnosis with doppler US. *Radiology*, **178**, 549–51

Index